GLOBESITY

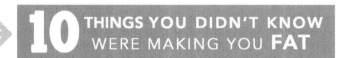

10 THINGS YOU DIDN'T KNOW
WERE MAKING YOU **FAT**

CLARE FLEISHMAN MS, RD

PLAIN SIGHT PUBLISHING

AN IMPRINT OF CEDAR FORT, INC.

SPRINGVILLE, UT

FOR JEFF

DISCLAIMER

The information provided in this book should not be used to diagnose or treat any medical condition. For diagnosis or treatment of any medical problem, consult your own physician. The publisher and author are not responsible for any specific health or allergy needs that may require medical supervision and are not liable for any damages or negative consequences from any treatment, action, application, or preparation, to any person reading or following the information in this book. References are provided for informational purposes only and do not constitute endorsement of any websites or other sources.

Although the author and publisher have made every effort to ensure that the information in this book was correct at press time, the author and publisher do not assume and hereby disclaim any liability to any party for any loss, damage, or disruption caused by errors or omissions, whether such errors or omissions result from negligence, accident, or any other cause.

ISBN 13: 978-1-4621-1296-8

Published by Plain Sight Publishing, an imprint of Cedar Fort, Inc.
2373 W. 700 S., Springville, UT 84663
Distributed by Cedar Fort, Inc., www.cedarfort.com

LIBRARY OF CONGRESS CATALOGING-IN-PUBLICATION DATA

Fleishman, Clare, 1955- author.
Globesity : 10 things you didn't know were making you fat / Clare Fleishman MS, RD.
  pages cm
Includes bibliographical references and index.
ISBN 978-1-4621-1296-8 (alk. paper)
1. Obesity. I. Title.

RA645.O23F565 2013
362.1963'98--dc23

  2013033028

Cover design by Angela D. Baxter
Cover design © 2013 by Lyle Mortimer
Edited and typeset by Whitney Lindsley

Printed in the United States of America

10 9 8 7 6 5 4 3 2 1

CONTENTS

· · · ·

INTRODUCTION

· · · ·

NOT FAR FROM THE NILE LIES A CANYON CALLED Wadi Degla. Its walls scratch the sky high above the desert floor, just as they have for millions of years. They make me feel young, these massive rocks carved from prehistoric oceans: me, with a mere half century stowed in Nike running shorts, zipping along in solitude beyond the dirt and noise of Cairo. I run here most days. I like the quiet, the deep shadows, the parched scrub, and the humbling sense that humans are specks on the evolutionary quilt. I like what it does for my head, and I really like what it does for my metabolism. My exercise in the heat allows me to eat more.

But I never burn as many calories as I'd like. There's never that sort of freedom; keeping trim is a battle with every bite, a struggle between need and desire. What does it take to maintain a healthy weight these days? Clambering up desert canyons seems to be one answer, at least for me. You'd think I'd have this diet and exercise loop down pat by now. I'm one of those people who knew every calorie and gram of carbohydrate, fat, and protein in any food, packaged or garden fresh. That obsession started when I was a teenager growing up in the United States, soon after the first weight bump hit and *Seventeen* magazine taunted me with anorexic images of highly paid waifs. It grew when I studied nutrition science in college and graduate school. There, at two research universities in the 1970s, from pioneers in a field that I'd had no clue was essentially in its infancy, I learned the Krebs cycle, the biochemical structure for all the vitamins, and the metabolic pathway for gluconeogenesis. I was amazed at how many vitamins and minerals and enzymes and coenzymes and nutrient factors were needed just to get a cookie to surrender its sugar. I knew this sophisticated stuff, but I also absorbed the banal: the percentage of vitamins leeched in boiled carrots (a lot); the reasons not to serve mashed potatoes with cauliflower and fish (hint: monochromatic equals unappetizing); and why refreezing raw meat is a bad idea (bacteria thrive).

I loved the science of nutrition. The more I learned, the more there was to learn. The human body was an infinite miracle of precision and wonder that would never divulge all its secrets. I especially liked the futuristic musings: the theories about using vitamins to prevent cancer, the hypothesis that chromium could somehow manage diabetes, and the notion that one of my nutrition professors swallowed niacin supplements to warm his toes on cold winter mornings. Nutrition would be the answer to heart disease, cancer, osteoporosis, and maybe even mental illness, once we figured out how to ford that stubborn blood-brain barrier. Surely obesity would be the easiest problem to figure out. Calories in and calories out would be simple math for us nutritionists.

I knew the Stillman and Atkins diets by heart. Unlimited bacon was one interesting kind of diet. Later while working as a registered dietitian, I carefully fashioned needs into nice 1200-1500-1800 calorie balanced menus. "Here you go," I'd tell my patients. "Here's your booklet and your twenty-minute instruction. Now go forth: lose weight, manage your diabetes, and reduce that cholesterol." I branched out. I took my message of good nutrition to locker rooms, radio stations, baby clinics, nursing homes, nursery schools, YMCAs, doctors' offices, transplant units, bypass units, synagogues, boardrooms, television news, high school assemblies, five-star kitchens, soup kitchens, psych hospitals, college cafeterias, food companies, diet companies, bridge clubs, newsrooms, Tupperware parties, and to lunch ladies, working moms, stay-at-home moms, weekend warriors, marathon men, and traveling salesmen. I never made it to a cruise ship, one unfortunate holdout on my list.

All across the modern landscape, armies of young dietitians like me lectured and cajoled day after day, year after year at hospitals, health fairs, schools, and pretty much anywhere there were people who ate. Somewhere along the way, though, other instructors of often-dubious credentials changed their names to health coaches and promised to reach deep inside their clients to understand and discover solutions to their weight problems. Obesity went prime time. Television viewers found the show *Biggest Loser* to be an instant winner; the not-so-little ones got help on BBC's *Too Fat to Toddle*; Rodale's *Men's Health* magazine went global, hitting newsstands in forty-seven countries, including Qatar, where rippled abs, hidden under crisp white tunics, see little sunlight. Diet books came and went, and then came back again: we mixed and matched and recycled high-protein, low-carbohydrate, low-fat, high-fat, and high-fiber menus and wrapped them in expensive zip codes such as Scarsdale, Beverly Hills, and South Beach. Losing weight could mean cabbage soup, baby food, raw food, juice cleanses, fake sugars, fake fats, all liquids, no foods, amphetamines, enemas, stapled stomachs, wired jaws, tongue patches, and much more. So how are we doing, thirty years later? You already know the answer.

Globesity.

Obesity plagues the globe. Starting with the United States, the ostensible ground zero for the problem, more than two-thirds of adults are overweight, and half of these are obese.[1] The epidemic sweeps far beyond American shores. The rest of the world is gaining too; for the first time in history, the number of overweight people has surpassed that of underweight.

The World Health Organization estimates that an astounding "1.4 billion adults [are] overweight"—almost one in three. What's more, "obesity rates have nearly doubled since 1980." And sadly, "more than 40 million children under the age of five are overweight."[2]

No corner of the planet is immune. Even in developing countries where people subsist on as little as two dollars a day, such as here in Egypt, where I live, obesity rates have skyrocketed. Broad beans called *fuul* and chewy *baladi* bread are the staples, just as they have been for centuries, yet the scales are groaning anyway. It is not uncommon to find undernutrition and obesity existing side-by-side within the same country, the same community, and even within the same plywood shanty.

Paradoxically, it is the rich who are fatter in the poorer,

developing countries, while the poor suffer more obesity in industrialized countries of Europe and the United States. It is a range that challenges health experts to tackle the epidemic from many angles.

Barefoot children beg for food when I shop in my neighborhood market; across the street, a doctor offers liposuction, the most popular cosmetic surgery in Egypt, a country of 83 million with a gross domestic product (GDP) the size of Tennessee's. Back in the United States, about 160,000 bariatric surgeries, which either band or cut most of the stomach pouch, were done in 2010.[3] Abandoning diets and exercise, some doctors prescribe surgery as the best way to get the weight off. Surgery, suctioning, and strong drugs are the drastic measures society has chosen. Traditional methods have failed miserably. Humans are fat and getting fatter.

As I trudge from rock to rock along the ancient Egyptian river bed, I ponder the obesity conundrum and wonder what it all means: if it even matters in the big picture, the one left frameless by the vast universe, the one which deems our significance as little more than lint. In other words, is obesity a problem worth solving? Does it kill more people than war or traffic accidents or malaria? What does it matter if people weigh too much—a few or forty or four hundred extra pounds. Maybe it doesn't matter.

But of course it does. A few or forty pounds—qualifying for the overweight but not yet obese category for most adults—may not kill you, but optimum health will be elusive. Still, a few groups are trying to get overweight people to accept their fate and go on with their lives. For some, that may be the best approach, especially when the battle devolves into eating disorders and mental problems. But unequivocally, the best health is impossible with excess weight. Hearts beat faster, colds last longer, breaths get shorter, and joints buckle under the strain. Good health depends on a strong body, unencumbered by the stress extra fat puts on our hearts, immune systems, lungs, stomachs, and every other part of our fragile yet resilient human bodies.

Obesity, on the other hand, can kill you: it is estimated that obesity causes hundreds of thousands of premature deaths in the United States alone.[4] And globally, nearly three million die early according to 2012 World Health Organization estimates.[5]

However, the risk of death from obesity depends on where a person falls in the obesity spectrum. A recent review of nearly a hundred studies concluded that lesser obesity or BMI below 35 was not linked with higher deaths.[6]

Obesity causes or worsens a slew of serious health problems, including cardiovascular disease, arthritis, gallbladder and kidney disease, and cancers of the breast, colon, uterus, esophagus, and kidneys. In the United States, direct and indirect costs of obesity could be as much as $147 billion each year, according to health economists.[7]

The enormous health impact of this obesity pandemic can be seen most clearly in fast-rising rates of type 2 diabetes, for which obesity is the main known risk factor. According to the Brussels-based International Diabetes Federation (IDF), the number of diabetics worldwide has grown to 371 million,[8] more than ten times what it was in 1985.[9] "The [IDF] predicts that unless rapid action is taken, one person in ten will have diabetes by 2030."[10]

Overnutrition kills as often as undernutrition; it just takes longer. Many thousands of people die from complications caused by obesity every year, though good statistics are elusive due to its place on the medical charts as a secondary diagnosis. It is more dignified to die from diabetes than obesity; sympathy is derived from a diabetic label even as obesity carries a taint of character weakness or individual blame. Yet in 2013, the American Medical Association has decided obesity is in fact a disease.

Most frightening is what has happened to our children. They are fat in record numbers. My childhood home in Pennsylvania is directly across from a school playground, one of the few that still attract small groups of kids in the summertime. During recent visits to see my family, I would sit on the front porch and watch as children of all ages trickled into the playground. My nutritionist's eye started seeing a pattern.

Time after time, my observations confirmed the statistics: a group of three little ones—one was overweight; a gang of six basketball players—two were heavier than they should be; a cluster of three preteen girls—maybe two were too large. And, most alarmingly, I realized that these were the kids who were out on the playground, not indoors watching television and eating potato chips. If I could peer beyond doors, I knew the scene would be even more disheartening.

Starting with the United States, epicenter of the pandemic, we see that the numbers of overweight children have more than tripled in the last three decades.[11] More than 10 percent of children worldwide are overweight according to the International Diabetes Federation.[12] Some countries claim more than their share: data from Wales show that 38 percent of boys ages 2 through 15 were overweight in 2012.[13] In oil-rich Kuwait, 40 to 46 percent of adolescents are estimated to be overweight or obese.[14] In India, just as in many other developing countries, obesity lives next door to hunger. A study conducted by the Delhi Diabetes Research Center among schoolchildren ages 10 to 16 found nearly one in five to be either overweight or clinically obese.[15] Yet figures from a National Family Health Survey revealed that in India "almost half of children under the age of [three] are underweight."[16] Most countries aren't as fastidious as India is about statistics. Global figures are often hard to come by. In the search for childhood obesity numbers, several factors obscure the count: stunting, which is caused by early malnutrition; different rates of sexual maturation; and errors in measurement.[17] But trends are unmistakable because the changes are coming so fast.

Beyond the emotional scars obesity inflicts on the playground—when overweight kids even dare venture there—are the diseases that go along with it. Kids are showing up in doctors' offices with kidney stones, high blood sugar levels, and blocked arteries. Boys are worrying about when to take their statin medication when they should be thinking about homework. Their medical records resemble a litany of troubles usually associated with middle age. This may very well be our pathetic legacy to our children: their generation may be the first in human history to have a shorter life expectancy than their parents. It is a frightening prospect and all because of excess weight and the damage it does.

I ponder this thought as a pale afternoon sun slips behind a towering limestone shelf in the canyon. I struggle up across the loose stones, sweating and panting like any woman intent on fighting the fat, that most formidable of foes. When I reach the summit, after I quiet my lungs, I drink in the view. On a rare day, I can see the great pyramids at Giza. But today is a typical day, one without that majestic view because the sky is choked with acrid smoke from burning trash, fumes from rotten exhaust pipes, and cement-particle clouds from factories. Incessant honking echoes in the distance. Unfinished apartment buildings in the Soviet bloc-design rim the perimeter. Poor Cairenes—they have enough problems. Now they can add obesity to the list.

Naturally I think about the pyramid we nutritionists know all too well. The Eating Right Pyramid, it turns out, is every bit as enigmatic as these stone wonders here in Giza. Nutrition experts kept changing it: adding blocks, narrowing categories, and chiseling portions until it became the new and improved United States Department of Agriculture (USDA) MyPyramid. In 2011, though, after 19 years of service, the pyramid was replaced. MyPlate became the official nutrition symbol. Maybe this one will stem the obesity epidemic.

I peer beyond a lip of rock into the canyon below; the path that threatened to trip me with rocks and gullies looks smooth from this vantage point as it ribbons its way through the valley. A Land Rover crawls along the path like a toy car, spitting up whorls of dust in its wake. The windows are closed, and I surmise the air-conditioning is running full-blast. I can't blame the driver. The air can be so thick it stings sometimes. I don't see many birds, though these *wadis* (Arabic for canyons) are supposed to be sanctuaries for them and foxes and other small wildlife. The pharaohs would not be pleased by the state of their modern Egypt. Sure, they'd like our twenty-first-century fast cars, fast food, and a world brought to their laps though the Internet. But the inconvenient truth about our easy living is becoming downright deadly.

Is our obesity pandemic just one more inconvenient truth? Maybe our environment, increasingly fouled from the steam and grit of the industrial revolution, is to blame.

Maybe the environment is making us fat.

No kidding, you may say, an environment teeming with deep-fried Snickers and excellent couch entertainment is absolutely an environment that makes us fat. No doubt about that. But are poor diets and lack of exercise the only reasons? Why is it so hard to lose weight? And why is it even harder to keep it off? Why do most people who lose weight regain it all five years later? Randomized controlled trials such as the Trials of Hypertension Prevention, Weight Loss Maintenance, PREMIER, the Women's Health Initiative dietary trial, and the Diabetes Prevention Program have shown that behavioral interventions can improve dietary patterns and physical activity levels, reduce body weight, lower blood pressure, reduce LDL levels, and prevent the onset of diabetes. The problem is that even the most successful behavioral change programs only result in temporary changes. Even participants most committed to making changes find it hard to maintain a healthy lifestyle over time. Most weight-loss studies show that after six months, participants begin to gain back lost weight, with a majority regaining all of the weight lost by five years.[18]

What can be done, if anything, to tackle this problem of epidemic proportions, to fight *globesity?*

We need to look beyond diet and exercise. Both are crucial solutions but not the only ones.

Imagine we all live in a petri dish called planet earth. For most of the 200,000 years humans have been around, their BMIs have stayed (except for gluttonous kings) within a healthy range of 20–21. But in the past thirty years, a few ticks on the clock of human existence, the percentage of BMIs in the overweight range (over 25) triples. It is an absolutely catastrophic event in the annals of science. A good scientist will look at the variables. What nutrition is sustaining them? Has it changed? Yes, certainly—from meat and potatoes to hormone-pumped burgers and trans fat-laden chips in just a few decades. Then she will ask: Are the organisms able to move? Yes, but it's not required of them to reach the nutrients. And then the good scientist announces: "That's it. I know why these organisms are fat." But the better scientist keeps looking. What else is different? Did someone contaminate the dish? What happened to the temperature of the milieu inside the dish? What else has changed that could be causing *globesity?*

Quite a lot has changed.

If melting tundra, sterile frogs, and dying fish are the havoc inflicted by our toxic environment, then perhaps—take the leap with me here—bulging waistlines, rising blood sugars, and proliferating fat cells are pieces of the iceberg we humans are seeing.

After my run, I slide into my *air-conditioned* Jeep Cherokee and flip on the radio which yields nothing but scratchy Arabic love songs. I pop in my iPod and crank it up to block out the *annoying honking* on the ride back to Maadi, a *suburb* of Cairo. Despite my best intentions and defensive driving efforts, I seethe and *swear* and generally undo all my good "running-in-the-canyon karma" on the obstacle course called an Egyptian highway: goats and donkeys, *wrong-way drivers*, whole families on motorbikes and car-sized craters are often the least of it. I yank my liter *plastic bottle* of Baraka water out of the cup holder and take a big gulp. A few meters past the mosque, I'm still a bit parched so I pull over at a fruit juice stand where a gallibayeed man with *dirt under his fingernails* squeezes a glass of strawberry-mango juice. Once at home, I immediately flip on my *computer* and try not to think about my expanding email inbox. I turn to the Middle East headlines. It's all too *depressing*. Maybe it's time to join the rest of the *Prozac* nation. Nah, a gooey dessert will be just as therapeutic.

Can you spot the toxins? My ten-minute ride home—universally average, except perhaps for the itinerant barnyard animal—threatened to undo all my good exercise and weight management efforts.

This book will take a look at some of these things, poisons in our petri dish called planet earth, and decide whether these are every bit as fattening as locking a kid in a candy store. Each chapter will look at the science—some of it in the social realm—and ask: could this be a contributor to the obesity epidemic? Some provocative research has already been published with scientists leading the way against a phalanx of traditionalists who want to put all the blame on the individual. One seminal paper written by a parade of obesity researchers entitled "Ten Putative Contributors to the Obesity Epidemic" points to obesogens including air-conditioning, medications, infections, and pollution.[19] This groundbreaking work was the seed for my book. As I investigated, the sweep of the evidence became apparent.

I'll take a deep look at the research, talk with scientists, and in the end explore how we can best eliminate or minimize the obesogenic effect of these other causes in our own lives.

I don't want to be right about this. I wish governments could solve it with a perfect nutrition pyramid or plate. I wish big pharma would design the perfect diet pill to dissolve fat, with absolutely no harmful side effects. I wish fad diet books would help readers lose weight, and keep it off. But I think this riddle is bigger than us now. The obesity epidemic threatens all of us, our children, and our grandchildren. It's time to attack it from a different angle.

Let's start with some unusual suspects. Here are ten to consider:

1. Air-conditioning
2. Medications
3. Pollution
4. Suburbs
5. Crime
6. Access
7. Contagions
8. Stress
9. Food additives
10. Sleep debt

When you look at the list and read the chapters ahead, you'll see that many are the very same ones that have laid waste to the planet's ecology. It sounds logical: why should humans be immune to poisons that sicken and kill other species? Polar bears are drowning without the safety of ice floes, brown bears are hibernating fewer months and starving when they awake to find berries still locked in their blossoms, frogs are disappearing forever, and humans are getting fatter. Obesity is just one more symptom of a very sick planet.

It's time to take control of our environments. It's time to quit sabotaging our best weight control efforts by ignoring the evidence. It's time to agree that green is lean.

1

. . . .

ADDICTED TO COOL:
AIR-CONDITIONING & OBESITY

Air-conditioning usage is exploding, right along with obesity rates.

MY FIRST JOB WITH A REAL PAYCHECK WAS counting cookie orders at a Nabisco distribution center in eastern Pennsylvania in 1971. It was the first summer of my life I spent indoors, sitting at a desk, stiff as a Popsicle—despite my wool sweater—in central air-conditioning. I gained ten pounds that summer. I can't prove it was the air conditioner; in fact, it never crossed my mind back then because there were other, more obvious reasons for my weight gain such as the endless supplies of Oreos and Triscuits from the warehouse. I returned to that frigid office for four more summers, collecting cookies, a paycheck, and the same ten pounds I had worked to take off the rest of the year.

I remember the earlier days when I swam and played volleyball and stayed outside most days, my arms beaded with sweat, my hair curly in the damp northeastern August. When I came home, I sat at the dinner table with little appetite for anything but ice water. Later in the evenings, my parents sat outside on the covered porch and played pinochle with neighbors until long after their eight young children were asleep beneath cool breezes from open windows. Fireflies danced across the lawns back then, and a majestic maple tree next to our sidewalk wrapped its branches and lush leaves around our house like a parasol; a striped awning did the rest.

Fast forward thirty-plus years: Air-conditioning is a fact of modern life. Wake up in an air-conditioned bedroom, hop into an air-conditioned SUV, stop by an air-conditioned Starbucks en route to the air-conditioned office, pump iron at the air-conditioned gym, drop by the air-conditioned mall, and then slide into the air-conditioned restaurant before hurrying to a film at the air-conditioned theater, after which head back to the air-conditioned house before starting it all over again the next day. How much of that hot summer day even slips through the cracks of our cool, cloistered lives?

Another fact of life today is obesity. As air-conditioning usage rates have skyrocketed, obesity rates have done the same. In countries as disparate as the United States, Saudi Arabia, China, and even tiny Nauru, an island in the South Pacific where 90 percent of the people are overweight, air-conditioning and obesity rates have climbed in tandem. Is it just a coincidence? The answer, sadly, is no. Investigations into the link between air conditioners and obesity have revealed alarming truths. A growing consensus exists among scientists that air-conditioning can contribute to obesity.

THE KINGDOM AND THE AMISH

Consider the Kingdom of Saudi Arabia. It may offer the quintessential evidence for the air-conditioning and obesity link. Here's why: It has modernized and grown fabulously wealthy in only a few decades. It has gone from a nation of tribal nomads to one of oil magnates, from a populace of movers to one of sitters, from a diet of beans and bread to McNuggets and Pepsi, and finally from a climate of hot, dry days to one of ubiquitous air-conditioned interiors. Because of these dramatic lifestyle changes in so short a time, the Kingdom presents us with the perfect microcosm to prove how obesity and air-conditioning are wed, though certainly fat is not limited to one partner.

The air-conditioning market in Saudi Arabia is growing at a brisk pace.[1] A visit to the capital city of Riyadh suggests that the LG electronics sales force has done its job very well, its mission for 100 percent market saturation close at hand. As in the United States, it is possible to spend an entire day—in a Saudi scorcher—in the thermoneutral zone (TNZ), the range where the body doesn't have to work to keep its temperature balance.[2] And, as in the United States, children and adults are finding they do not want to go outdoors to be uncomfortable. People are now acclimatizing to cooler temperatures. Indoors, of course, the activities are much more sedentary and food is just steps away. And to no one's surprise, Saudi children are obese.[3, 4] The King Faisal Specialist Hospital is overloaded with obesity-related problems and is seeing severe health problems in young people normally associated with adults: hypertension, diabetes, arthritis, and back ailments.[5]

A number of members from the ruling family House of Saad have journeyed to weight management camps, such as one in the countryside near the Old Order Amish settlements in Pennsylvania. The camps teach portion control—rather, they impose it—and sports participation; they have a full schedule of tennis, basketball, swimming, and anything else a college campus offers. Most days are spent outdoors in the muggy northeastern climate, a steam bath that can be worse than the scorching dry heat of a desert homeland. In camp, the Saudi kids eat healthy food like fruit salads, raw vegetables, and yogurt dip dished up in a cafeteria as they learn to live without plates of brownies and sodas delivered by household servants. Group sessions offer discussions of "food issues" and dietitians teach healthy cooking, lessons perhaps lost on kids who never before stepped inside a kitchen. Most lose a lot of weight. Then they return to their pampered environment and the weight is put back on.

Meanwhile, down the road from the camp, young girls in prim dresses and bonnets and little boys in long pants and straw hats tend to chores on an Amish farm: tilling fields, feeding pigs and chickens, baking bread, and shelling beans for dinner. For fun, the "plain folk"—which the Amish prefer to be called—ride bikes and chase cows in the fields; school is in a simple room near their homes, a throwback to television's *Little House on the Prairie*. The community eschews electricity, which means no computers, televisions, or air conditioners. Now take a look at Amish obesity rates: 0 percent for men and just 9 percent for women.[6] Twenty-five percent of these men and 29 percent of women fall into the overweight category with BMIs above 25, both groups far leaner than the not-so-plain folk they see in air-conditioned cars on the way to air-conditioned shopping malls.

Amish people, especially the men, expend an incredible amount of energy in the farm fields. Their menus resemble those of our grandparents, before Cheetos and Pop Tarts invaded pantries. This means lots of fresh fruits and vegetables but with generous portions of meat and potatoes. While growing up in Pennsylvania, I often enjoyed their culinary treats, such as gooey shoofly pie and doughy soft pretzels. Evidently, the Amish are not eating Lean Cuisine to maintain those figures.

Exercise accounts for much of the difference. And, undeniably, the Amish don't use air-conditioners. Except for penchants for female hair coverings, Saudi Arabian and Amish cultures could not be more different. Unlike the Saudi children, Amish children prefer playing outdoors, even on the hottest of summer days, when heat indexes rival desert temperatures. Indoors for the plain folk provides no cool rooms and big-screen televisions. Instead they search for cool breezes under weeping willows or a splash in a small pond. After chores, that is. But even if intense heat were to make them lazy, more inclined to nap under that tree, their bodies would still be burning more energy at rest. See, heat makes extra work for the body. Air-conditioning removes that job—a job requiring calories—which we humans have had to do since we started walking upright. Granted, heat can be insufferable in a Saudi desert. And shade trees and ponds may be scarce in the Saudi desert. But the dependence on air-conditioning may prove to be a less-than-perfect solution.

How large of a factor is air-conditioning in obesity, given that so much in modern life has changed? It is difficult to measure exactly, but we can use science to come up with good estimates. But first, let's take a closer look at air-conditioning and its startling spread across the globe, even in the poorest of countries.

SHORT STORY OF AIR-CONDITIONING

Air-conditioning makes us comfortable. It's tough to argue with comfort, especially when it involves chilling in front of a wide-screen plasma television and Xbox 360. Unfortunately, the human body has not yet adapted to the luxury climate control and sedentary pleasures that the last few decades have afforded. For the 200,000 years of human history, we have had to expend extra energy to contend with frigid cold and hellacious hot. Earth's earliest humans lived in sub-Saharan Africa, where they were able to survive the brief winters and long summers. They began migrating about 65,000 years ago to southern Asia and later Spain and Italy. Cold weather was a challenge. Rubbing two sticks together solved some of the problem, as anyone could sit near a wood fire to wait out the meanest storm, if there was shelter from a cave or other dry spot. Eventually fossil fuels were discovered: coal could burn longer and throw off as much heat as wood. Patterns of human migration show that the earliest communities were better able to survive hot climates than cold.

Huge blocks of ice became the earliest refrigerants. By keeping food cold, people in the 1800s avoided diseases from salmonella and *E. coli*. Massive slabs of ice cut from Fresh Pond near Harvard College and protected by sawdust and blankets were heaved onto train cars in Boston and sent all the way to Calcutta in India. Ice-houses were also built in Charleston and New Orleans to help cool the South in the early 1900s.[7]

That all changed when a young man named Willis Carrier designed the world's first air-conditioner, essentially a refrigerator without the box to hold food. In 1902, he installed his creation for a publishing company in Brooklyn, New York. Madison Square Gardens, the United States Senate, department stores, and corporations all lined up for this new technology. One in particular, the Johnson Wax Building in Racine, Wisconsin, designed by Frank Lloyd Wright in 1936 to be almost completely devoid of windows—thus making air-conditioning a necessity—was ridiculed by Henry Miller in his 1970 essay "The Air-Conditioned Nightmare."[8] Even so, business was brisk on the commercial front until the Depression and World War II turned the public's attention to more pressing matters.

Post-war America brought a whole new set of clients, according to Adam Rome, author of *The Bulldozer in the Countryside*.[9] Sales of room units went from 43,000 in 1947 to over one million by 1953, largely as a result of clever marketing to both wives and builders.

Men, it was assumed, were already sold on the concept because they worked in air-conditioned offices. Hence women were targeted with a no-fail sales pitch: air-conditioning would improve family life. It would offer sounder sleep, less dust indoors, more comfortable play-time for the kids, and a better sociable ambience for evening parties. Few wives could resist the lure of such promise, a box that has now proved more Pandoran than palliative.

The customers wanted it, if only they could afford it. So to absorb the cost of adding air conditioners, home builders were persuaded by the cooling industry to cut corners. Which they did, literally. Ranch-style hot boxes were the result. Without architectural features like breezeways, porches, basements, screened-in sleeping porches, and with fewer cross-ventilating windows and mature trees, this modern home relied on electric-powered air-conditioning to provide relief in hot weather, a seasonal irritant for much of the United States, which had traditionally been confronted by good environmental design. The next challenge for the air-conditioning industry was to design units and technology that would make air-conditioning in cars both small and affordable. They succeeded: it is a rare vehicle that comes off an assembly line today without a cooling system, according to the Air-Conditioning and Refrigeration Institute. It is no longer an expensive option for the consumer; it is now included in the base price. Even countries with cool climates most of the year, such as Britain, took to the luxury of chilled transport: today more than 75 percent of new cars have air-conditioning.

Willis Carrier had succeeded: today the Carrier Company employs "nearly 61,000 employees operating in more than 170 countries on six continents."[10] Homes built with central air, accord-ing to the Air-Conditioning and Refrigeration Institute, have risen significantly in the last 30 years (36 to 87 percent).[11] Most of the older homes built in the years before the necessary ductwork was constructed have at least one room air-conditioner. Many use five or six to cool all the bedrooms and living spaces. Public indoor spaces are air-conditioned, nearly 100 percent in the United States. In European countries, department stores and corporate buildings have followed suit, but at a much slower pace than in the United States. American tourists in Italy and Spain find the lack of air-conditioning appalling, yet these Mediterranean countries had long handled the heat with afternoon siestas.

Americans use more energy for air-conditioning than the rest of the world combined. That sad fact comes courtesy of scientist Stan Cox, author of *Losing Our Cool: Uncomfortable Truths About Our Air-Conditioned World (and Finding New Ways To Get Through the Summer)*. Cox writes: "In fact, we use more electricity for cooling than the entire continent of Africa, home to a billion people, consumes for all purposes. Between 1993 and 2005, with summers growing hotter and homes larger, energy consumed by residential air-conditioning in the U.S. *doubled*, and it leaped another 20 percent by 2010."[12]

Energy consumption is only one of the downsides. Another, possibly even more egregious problem is what spews out from these boxes: hot air and carbon dioxide—as much as 40 percent of the energy is wasted—which contributes enormously to global warming. On a local scale, it raises the outside temperature of the cities, whose inhabitants then crank up the air, which then creates more heat, thus creating a positive feedback loop, or a vicious cycle depending on which side of the Carrier transaction you happen to be on. Blackouts have been common in recent heat waves. Electrical grids of major cities such as New York and Mumbai cannot meet the demand.

I don't want to demonize air-conditioning. In fact, air conditioners have saved many lives. Look at the thousands of elderly people in Paris who died from dehydration and heat stroke in the summer of 2003 when temperature and humidity beat the charts for weeks on end. Their cramped apartment block buildings weren't designed for those temperatures in the same way as Roman apartments, where marble floors and high ceilings and vast windows are the norm for summer cooling. Perhaps that sad accident of climate for the French will be seen as a one-off or it may become more familiar, with global warming on the march as it is. In another vein, how many surgeries would be as successful without air-conditioning? Surgeons will not do their best work with sweat running down their brows after standing in heat for long hours. In addition to the cooling effect, operating room air is also filtered to reduce infection and the humidity controlled to limit patient dehydration. And don't forget this: how many computers would overheat and crash without the optimum temperatures provided by air-conditioning? This last may be the real reason for the rampant rise in indoor cooling. The tools of technology are fragile. They require a whole new set of creature comforts.

Now we need air-conditioning. The proof is in our enormous productivity: work never has to stop. Studies have shown that people seated in an office work best at 72°F (22°C). Performance is said to degrade about 1 percent for every 2°F change in temperature. Slightly lower temperatures are optimum for larger workers and people who are standing.

Countries closer to the equator are getting the message: with the hum of air-conditioning in offices, those traditional afternoon naps at home will be history. Nevertheless, one such country, Italy, could make the argument that Michelangelo and his siesta-taking contemporaries did a pretty good job for the economy, even without the cool comfort of air-conditioning. Today, treasures like the Sistine Chapel in Rome are cooled by Carrier units.

China and the rest of the world are following in the heavy carbon footprint of the United States. Demand in China has tripled since the year 2000, according to a report from the Freedonia Group, Inc., a Cleveland-based market research firm. *The Economist* magazine reports that "between 1995 and 2004 the proportion of homes in Chinese cities with air-conditioning rose from 8 percent to 70 percent."[13]

In summer, the air-conditioners in China require a sapping 40 percent of the country's electrical supply. Two-thirds of this electricity is coal-fired, which explains why dense black smog suffocates many of China's big cities.[14] Global sales rose 13 percent in 2011 from the year before, and that is expected to accelerate in coming decades, according to Cox.[15]

A stroll through an average Cairo neighborhood reveals the predominant five- to ten-story concrete apartment dwellings. These belong to the middle classes (the poorest must settle for frond shacks in this city without rain). While more often than not the walls in the tall buildings are crumbling and the windows are dirty, few are without the modern necessities of life: satellite dishes and air-conditioning units. Egypt is not a country known for precise statistics, but even casual observation tells a story of an exploding number of units. In the Middle East demand for room air conditioners has doubled since 2000, according to industry reports. Where there is electricity, there is a way.

AIR-CONDITIONING AND OBESITY

Air-conditioning rates mirror the alarming growth in obesity around the world. The growing scientific consensus is that air-conditioning can contribute to obesity. How, exactly, is this possible?

First, air-conditioning affects how much we eat, or the energy coming in.

Second, air-conditioning affects how many calories we burn, or the energy going out.

Air-conditioning assaults the energy equation from both sides. Energy coming in must equal energy going out for a body to stay the same weight. Unfortunately, air-conditioning both increases the energy in and decreases the energy out so that the equation looks very lopsided. Let's take a look at how this works.

Energy In

One hot summer day, David Allison, professor of biostatistics at the University of Alabama in Birmingham, told *Bloomberg News*: "Yesterday in Alabama, it was 100 degrees; if you were here in 1960, with no air-conditioning in a car or restaurant, you probably wouldn't want to go to an all-you-can-eat buffet." Evidently not. In one consumer survey, restaurant sales dropped dramatically after an air-conditioner broke.[16] Customers were not very hungry. Why do you think we're forced to take a sweater to Applebee's? Consumer science is just that—a science. Applebee's management knows that people are going to order more ribs if they're a little chilled than if they are perspiring.

But why? Why don't we want to eat so much when it's hot? Are we just too sapped to lift the fork, or is it nature's way of protecting us? The simplest answer is that a lot of food just isn't appealing when we're sweating. Hot cocoa looks downright unpleasant when the mercury is over 90 degrees; but watermelon, a wedge plump with water, is enticing. However, the *reason* our taste buds are finicky is much more complex.

In hot weather, people sweat to cool the body. The acidity of the blood changes and as a result, gastric digestive juices decline. The blood supply flowing to the gut falls because more blood is shunted to the skin surface. Also, less saliva is available for digestion. All of these combine to shrink appetite and keep hunger pangs at bay. Both animal and human studies show that excursions above the thermoneutral zone markedly reduce food intake. The sweat and saliva changes are just two of the ways that happens. Some of the best questions have been asked by researchers working in the dairy industry; it seems that heat has a profound impact on milk production. As it turned out, I didn't have to look too far from my hometown to find some answers.

The Penn State Creamery scoops up tons of ice cream in fun flavors every year but none more popular than plain vanilla, which sells particularly well on football Saturdays in Happy Valley, as the 50,000 students prefer to call their college setting. Not far from campus, out along rural roads with numbers instead of names, cows graze the green-carpeted farmlands of central Pennsylvania. While ice cream may be these cows' sweetest contribution, the herds have also supplied reams of valuable data for the Penn State Dairy and Animal Science Department. Scientists here find research grants easy to get because anything that will fill milk cartons faster is likely to interest the government and dairy industry. Heat and humidity, which can get pretty thick in the northeast summers, wither the herds. This setting has given scientists much of the valuable information on what heat stress does to mammals.

Under normal conditions, cows use conduction and convection (non-evaporative methods of radiation) to get rid of excess heat. As heat gets more intense, though, the cow has to pant and sweat to channel some of the heat through water (evaporative). But if it's too humid, the cows cannot dissipate enough heat to prevent the rise in core temperature. So what do they do? They don't eat as much, which in turn reduces heat creation. The farmer wouldn't mind that so much, except for the stingy milk yield that goes along with it. As a result, the dairy farmer has learned a few things to keep profits churning.

One method is to fool the cow by increasing nutrient density of the feed; think Ensure Plus for the bovine set. But it is one thing to fool the eye yet quite another to fool the stomach, or stomachs in a cow's case.

The very best way to keep that milk flowing, farmers have found, is to prevent the problem of heat stress by keeping the cow cool. Methods include providing shade, adding fans and sprinklers, and building specially designed barns that encourage passive ventilation.

In a 2003 *Journal of Dairy Science* review article on heat stress in cattle, the author wrote that "maintaining cow performance in hot, humid climactic conditions in the future will likely require improved cooling capability, continued advances in nutritional formulation, and the need for genetic advancement which includes selection for heat tolerance."[17]

Cows are performing phenomenally. Milk yield in the industry has doubled in recent years, thanks to climate control, better nutrition, and smart matchmaking—tall, hot, and Holstein did the trick. However, the increases in growth and milk make heat production even greater.[18] Fortunately, when the cow is cooled sufficiently, her appetite returns.

Enough about cows. What about the millions of rodents that have sacrificed to illuminate the human struggle—what have we learned from them about temperature and obesity? Quite a bit, it turns out. Because rats share many of the same genes as humans, they have been used extensively to study obesity, diabetes, and even mental disorders such as schizophrenia. And since rats are cheaper, don't live as long as cows, and seem to be in limitless supply, research has a quicker turnaround time. It seems the rats react to heat in a similar fashion as cows: they don't eat as much. And with rats we have a clearer window on "why." *Rattus norvegicus*, a common lab rat, is sufficiently similar to humans in that it has hormones such as insulin and corticosterone. Researcher couple Lois and Theodore Zucker bred a special pair of rats called the Zucker rats, one lean and one genetically obese. In one experiment, scientists put both types of rats in 22°C (room temperature or 72°F) or 30°C (hot or 86°F) temperatures. The obese rats that by genetic design usually eat excessively—a condition called hyperphagia—ate less when the temperature rose. So did the lean ones.[19]

Insulin levels were studied in an experiment at Louisiana State University, a locale well known for its steamy summers. The ability of "timed daily increases" in ambient temperature was shown to decrease obesity in male Holtzman rats in part by "decreasing plasma insulin levels apparently as a consequence of increased tissue sensitivity to insulin." Insulin worked better in the heat.[20]

Pigs too are unfortunate to be similar enough to humans to be chosen research subjects. The influence of temperature on food intake was studied in piglets weaned at two weeks and kept in either 35°C (hot or 95°F) or 10°C (cool or 50°F) on various caloric intakes. Food intake was much greater in the cold than in the heat. Surprisingly, long-term cold had a lasting effect on the piglets' food intake even after they were back in normal temperatures. The authors surmised this outcome to be caused by hormonal changes.[21]

Two studies conducted at the University of Maastricht in the Netherlands put human subjects in respiration chambers at different temperatures and observed energy intake. The same phenomenon was observed as was seen in cows, rats, and pigs: humans ate more in cooler temperatures.[22]

Appetite. A simple word but a staggeringly complex phenomenon. Appetite is the desire to eat food. Hunger, on the other hand, is the pure physiological drive for food. Without appetite or hunger, a mammal doesn't eat and eventually dies. So, noting the supreme importance of eating, higher species regulate this desire by an exquisite signaling system involving the brain, gastrointestinal tract, fat tissue, organs, and hormones.

In the brain, the hypothalamus acts as a command center, weaving messages about energy coming in, energy going out, and energy being stored. The hypothalamus is bombarded with input from the mouth, the liver, the digestive tract, and even other parts of the brain. These messages take the form of hormones, such as insulin, leptin, and ghrelin, as well as chemicals named neuropeptide Y and Agouti-related peptide. There are doubtless other shadowy players that have yet to be identified. Once the master plan is set in motion, a person feels hunger, eats, feels satisfied, and ultimately stops until the hunger pangs start up again, about four hours later. When the plan is working perfectly, the amount eaten is exactly the amount necessary to maintain a healthy weight, a set point that veers little from day to day, or year to year.

But many factors can throw off the plan or override the precision: emotions such as boredom or sadness can make a person eat more, or less; visual cues such as being offered a piece of Godiva chocolate even after a filling lunch; exercise before a meal kills the appetite; consuming big portions for a long period make it more difficult to satisfy an appetite; and after just two weeks of a high-fat diet, the body adapts by digesting and storing fat more efficiently. And as was seen in cows, rats, and pigs, temperature will affect appetite in humans.

How temperature does this requires a brief introduction to some of the performers in the appetite game: leptin, neuropeptide Y, ghrelin, and insulin. A mouthful, for sure, yet all are crucial in appetite control, either by stoking it or choking it.

Let's start with leptin, whose story has been a cautionary tale for the multibillion-dollar obesity industry. Back in 1994, when researchers at The Rockefeller University in New York City identified leptin, a hormone secreted from white fat cells, many thought it would be the magic bullet for obesity. Mice lacking leptin ate greedily and grew obese; leptin injections cut their appetites and their weight. Eureka! The scientists who discovered leptin were probably thinking Nobel prizes. Unfortunately, humans turned out to react very differently. Scientists found that most obese people had lots of leptin; it just wasn't working the way it should, which is to signal the hypothalamus to slow down the appetite and speed up the metabolism. A flurry of research followed the discovery. One team of researchers correlated low leptin levels to weight gain in Pima Indians, a community with high obesity levels. But subsequent studies found either no relationship or an opposite result: higher leptin levels predicted more weight gain.[23] It appears that obese people may be leptin-resistant, or leptin-insensitive. This is a similar scenario to how insulin relates to diabetes. A type 2 diabetic has a pancreas that secretes enough insulin to deliver sugar to cells, but those target cells are rolling up the welcome mat.

The leptin star has dimmed. People aren't lining up for injections. But don't count it out completely. Its effects are turning up across the constellation of substances that figure in energy balance. For example, leptin is also thought to regulate insulin secretion and regulation of insulin action. And it is well established that insulin plays a major part in regulating appetite. Moreover, leptin works by manipulating neurotransmitters. One is called neuropeptide Y (NPY); small doses of NPY injected into his brain make an animal eat more. In a Canadian study, NPY was shown to affect body temperature and food intake. Body temperature and calorie intake are drastically altered at extreme temperatures. "In comparison with [more moderate] ambient temperatures of 12 and 21°C [54°F and 70°F], ambient temperatures of 4 and 30°C [39°F and 86°F] significantly reduced the stimulatory effect of NPY on food consumption." So at high temperatures, NPY was not increasing food consumption as it normally does. Clearly, when the mercury rose, NPY took a nap: the result was a smaller appetite.[24]

Ghrelin is a hormone that tells us to eat more. Isolated by Japanese researchers in 1999, ghrelin is made in the stomach and small intestine. Ghrelin increases food intake by activating NPY. Like a worried mom, ghrelin jumps into action after we lose a few pounds. It's no wonder it is so hard to keep weight off.

Cortisol is also emerging as a direct stimulator of leptin. Most people recognize this hormone as a stress hormone. When it is secreted in the body after a stressful situation, cortisol speeds up the breakdown of fat and proteins and thus raises blood sugar. Air-conditioning affects cortisol. Researchers at Fukuoka Women's University in Japan studied the influence of the long-term use of air-conditioning in summer on cortisol rhythms. Those exposed for a long period in September compared to those exposed in July had delayed morning cortisol secretion.[25] Even though these researchers were studying cortisol in relation to sleep habits, the results are relevant because cortisol also affects leptin, that stealthy arbiter of appetite. Simply put, cool air temperature decreases cortisol, which in turn decreases leptin, which in turn increases appetite. Connect the dots: air conditioners are making us fat by disturbing normal metabolic and hormonal rhythms of the body. And that is only after we're born.

The womb, in fact, is the first environment that sets up the new human being to be fat or thin. Numerous studies show that if a woman eats too little or smokes during pregnancy, her child is more likely to be fat or grow into an overweight adult. Our bodies are programmed even before we are born to struggle for nutrients in a harsh environment. The so-called "thrifty gene" continues to salivate even when times aren't so tough anymore, such as after birth, when a menu of unlimited food beckons. Now we can add air-conditioning to the list of no-no's when a woman is expecting. One interesting study done at Pennington Biomedical Research Center in Baton Rouge, Louisiana, tested the hypothesis that prenatal ambient temperature alters sympathetic activity in rats and affects body composition in adult rats. From one week before birth, rat litters were raised at either 18°C (cool or 64°F) or 30°C (hot or 86°F) until 2 months of age. The rats were then provided either a high-fat or low-fat diet. The rats reared in cool temperatures gained more weight on both diets than those reared in higher temperatures. Indeed, prenatal temperature affects body weight in rats.[26] Our bodies pack an inspiring mélange of weapons to make sure we don't starve. Because we have evolved from hunter-gatherers when food was not always a few steps away, humans who survived had superior genetic ammunition to induce hunger (leptin, ghrelin, and many others, some not yet discovered) when fat stores inside their bodies were running low or when a source of food like lion meat became available. As obesity researcher Rudolph Leibel of Columbia University told *The Economist*: "The evolutionary process has led to a gene pool that is designed to defend body weight against falling below a minimum, but not to defend against gain."[27]

Today, when food is not only available 24/7 but is also dense in fat and sugar, the body has little need of these appetite stokers. Our painstakingly-evolved tools for survival now threaten us.

Energy Out

The flip side of the equation is how air-conditioning affects energy being spent. Air-conditioning reduces calorie expenditure. It does this in several ways; one is more obvious such as enticing kids to stay indoors where they can't run around. But air-conditioning also outsources an important job, one we won't want to lose.

Whether on a hot day in summer or a visit to the sauna, our bodies work to adjust to the peril of high temperatures. We are not as lucky as reptiles and other exothermic animals whose body temperatures change with the weather. We are endothermic. This means we must work to keep a close watch on 37°C (98.6°F) or suffer the loss of limb or life. Our bodies manage the heat budget—a process called thermoregulation—so that the rate of heat gain equals the rate of heat loss. Remember the mantra for our physical selves: energy in must equal energy out. But what is the ultimate purpose of this adaptive means of maintaining an optimum temperature? The reason our bodies work so hard is to protect our core temperature so that vital organs are spared. In a blizzard, for example, the body is willing to sacrifice less important appendages like toes and fingers, to send heat inward to the heart and liver. The reverse, heat shuttled to the skin and beyond, is true in a heat wave. It's Physiology 101: Increased blood flow to the skin or vasodilation warms the skin and decreased blood flow or vasoconstriction cools the skin. This simple science belies the magical intelligence by which our bodies automatically jump into survival mode when threatened, in this case by extreme temperatures.

Other tricks from the Darwinian bag kick in to adjust the rate of heat exchange between an organism and its environment. In humans, for instance, insulation such as fat below the skin and hair on top reduces outward heat flow, protecting from a cold environment. In animals, within days or weeks in a cold environment, fur or fat insulation will accelerate. One creative study done at University of California, Berkeley measured energy intake for two to three weeks after hamsters had been completely shaved. They concluded, "Increases in food intake varied with condition and were greater in hamsters housed . . . at low . . . ambient temperatures."[28]

Modern man boasts less body hair than his cave-dwelling ancestors. We simply don't need it (or want it, if Brazilians have anything to say about it). The advent of fire as a heat source made hairy torsos obsolete. These mechanisms of acclimatization may also be at work when a human is put in an air-conditioned environment. If rats will compensate by adding fur and fat, humans perhaps have retained some of their own ability from long ago, a vestige of prehistory. Our talent for storing fat was once a lifesaver; these days, it's a killer.

Another survival technique is cooling by evaporative loss, such as perspiration, whereby heat is carried by water to the outside. And yet another adaptation to extreme temperatures—keeping the core organs functioning properly is worth so much to survival that evolution has come up with many alternate solutions if one is not enough—is by changing behaviors: moving about in the cold or shivering to maintain heat. These require energy.

And finally there are differences in metabolic heat production. For example, in hot climates, humans can tolerate a rise in body heat from the normal 37°C (98.6°F)—this enhances heat loss by increasing the temperature gradient between the body and a warm environment. And here comes the part where we loop back to how air-conditioning contributes to obesity: Thermoregulation requires energy. In some instances, the adaptation to heat stress requires blood flow away from another area of the body. The very act of regulating heat or thermoregulation is no longer needed when humans cool the atmosphere artificially. The heat stressors of the summer months are no longer present. No calories are used.

Simply put, humans make heat whether they are moving or sitting at a desk. This heat leaves easily when temperature outside is about 72°F or room temperature. As thermometers rise and get closer to body temperature of 98.6°F, the body has to work harder—like wrestling its own weight—to get rid of the heat. We use energy. Thus, the more time humans spend in a climate-controlled environment (air-conditioning in the heat of the summer), the less their bodies have to work. It is no coincidence that as childhood obesity rates have become epidemic—tripling in two decades in the United States—habits have also changed from the summers of my youth. Children growing up in the 1950s and 1960s spent much of their time outdoors in the summer. Weight gained during the winter months (rooted in evolutionary imperatives) was lost in the frenzied activity of summer. Today the opposite is true. Children gain more weight during the summer months. Recent research from Ohio State University tracked five thousand children from 990 schools as they traveled through kindergarten and first grade. The result?

"Children gain body mass index (BMI) nearly twice as fast during the summer as during the school year."[29] Likewise, a study from the University of Wisconsin Children's Hospital showed unhealthy changes during the three-month summer break. Overweight middle school children participated in a fitness intervention group for a full school year (roughly nine months). Improvements seen during the nine-month intervention as measured by cardiovascular fitness, fasting insulin levels, and body composition were lost during the three-month summer break.[30] In another example, more than 400 children in Tokyo were tracked by the Japanese National Institute of Public Health in six waves between 1972 and 2004. Each child's weight was measured monthly for six years. The authors concluded, "Weight gain in the summer was observed exclusively among obese children. Children whose weight increased during the summer holiday spent most of their time comfortably indoors because of air conditioners, which became popular [there] in the 1970s."[31]

Thus it is no longer possible to simply blame schools with their junk food and lack of physical education for our childhood obesity epidemic. Reasons for the seasonal changes are the following: energy expenditure is down because children are kept indoors, where it is cool and crime-free; food is more accessible inside; appetite increases due to cooler indoor temperatures; and the lack of heat stress effects appetite and energy expenditure as a result of air-conditioning.

In 1981, only one in three American households with central air used it all summer long. By 1997, more than half did. "The best attribute of air-conditioning is its addiction," said a marketing chief for LG electronics.[32] The *Economist* magazine reported that "Gwyn Prins, a Cambridge University professor, called 'physical addiction' to cooled air America's 'most pervasive and least noticed epidemic.'"[33]

Is air-conditioning addicting?

In a sense, yes. Just as nicotine, one of the most addictive substances in existence, changes the chemistry of our bodies, so does air-conditioning.

How that happens is well explained by science. Climbers tackling the world's highest mountains must acclimatize to survive a summit and then to get back down—the most dangerous part—when the weather can change in a minute. Acclimatization is an amazing process by which organisms adapt to new temperatures, altitudes, climates, or situations. Many plants such as tomatoes can survive freezing temperatures if the temperature gradually drops lower and lower each night over a period of days or weeks. The same drop might kill them if it occurred suddenly. Tropical fish likewise need a gradual change in temperature to get used to the home aquarium, but they can eventually thrive.

Researchers wrote in a 2006 issue of *Journal of Dairy Science* that

> Substantial progress has been made in the last quarter-century in delineating the mechanisms by which thermal stress and photoperiod influence performance of dairy animals. Acclimation to thermal stress is now identified as a homeorhetic process under endocrine control. The process of acclimation occurs in 2 phases (acute and chronic) and involves changes in secretion rate of hormones as well as receptor populations in target tissues. The time required to complete both phases is weeks rather than days.[34]

This means that the body adjusts when confronted with high temperatures. Basal metabolic rate and heart rate both increase in heat, thus expending more energy. Yet adaptation or acclimatization kicks in and the body learns to cool down. What is the takeaway message? Basically, if we put up with a little initial discomfort, our bodies will adapt to make us more comfortable. If we don't switch on the air on the first hot day in summer, we won't need as much. Our metabolisms and the environment both benefit.

Here's a "which came first, chicken or the egg" question: Does poor dissipation of heat contribute to obesity? Or is it the other way around—does obesity contribute to deficient heat dissipation? Either way, air-conditioning jumps into the fray. When ongoing clinical studies give us more answers on the temperature and obesity link, we will be able to fit this piece into the puzzle.

Another issue to consider is that the temperatures of homes, offices, and public buildings are rarely within our control. Think about it. Have you ever had the optimum indoor temperature debate with your mother, your husband, or your boss? Well, probably not with your boss if you valued your job. But thinking back to those high school summers when I worked in the Nabisco office, I realized the chocolate-coated Mystic Mints would melt in warm temperatures. But then so would the overweight people sitting near me. I was adapting to their comfort needs—because they could not dissipate heat properly, which was either a cause or effect of obesity. At first I wore a sweater and shivered, but then gradually I warmed up by eating more. By the end of the summer, I was switching on the air conditioner when I got home because I could no longer tolerate heat. I had very efficiently acclimatized—to cold indoor air in the middle of summer. My supervisors were spreading their obesogenic habits, a phenomenon observed by scientists at the Framingham Heart Study, who observed that obesity travels in social groups. I've known many people who handled heat poorly. Some were evidently addicted to air-conditioning because they were always in it. Others were, I suspect, victims of provenance. What temperature was their first environment, the womb? Is month of birth—cold and snowy January as opposed to steamy August—important, or have heating and air systems turned that theory on its ear? Does it matter if a Dubliner moves to Florida or if a Kenyan moves to Alaska? Why are so many more Hispanic women in the United States overweight than white women of European descent who live next door? It could be that their Hispanic ancestors, born into the considerable heat of countries like Puerto Rico and Mexico, have passed down their thrifty genes, those genes with instructions to save calories to meet demands of heat stress. When thrust into a place where heat stress is vanquished by a Carrier unit, where those once lifesaving thrifty genes are no longer needed or wanted yet are still ruling the appetite, could it be *then* that they become obese?

This line of thinking is already being investigated in the dairy industry. The newest ideas revolve around genetic selection of cows that don't mind heat as much and keep on eating and making milk.

Individual metabolisms are very different. In 2012 Dutch researchers at Maastricht University suggested that large differences exist between individuals in adaptive thermogenesis to cold or diet. This could explain why some people are more likely to become obese than others: "*Other* mechanisms besides mitochondrial uncoupling that might be involved are futile calcium cycling, protein turnover, and substrate cycling. In conjunction with recent advances on signal transduction studies, this knowledge makes manipulation of adaptive thermogenesis a more realistic option and thus a pharmacologically interesting target to treat obesity."[35]

In other words, the search is on for more magic pills, aka drugs. Another way to tackle the differences would be to teach those souls with poor adaptive thermogenesis skills to stay in the kitchen even if they can't stand the heat. Like the tropical fish, they may need more time to physiologically adapt, but they will.

It's time to rethink our romance with air-conditioning. It's bad for the environment and it's contributing to globesity.

Many summer issues of shelter magazines—magazines focused on interior design, home furnishing, and so on—offer tips on keeping cool naturally. Successful cooling strategies are similar to those mentioned earlier for cows: convection, conduction, radiation, and evaporation. Air movement with fans, wetting the cow's body surface, high pressure mist to cool the air in the cows' environment, and facilities designed to minimize the transfer of solar radiation are used.

SOLUTIONS

Trust your body to adapt when temperatures rise. These techniques will make warm weather tolerable while allowing your body to do its job of keeping you cool:

1. Insist on good environmental design. This works only for people who may be buying a new home or remodeling an old one. Request that architectural features like breezeways, porches, screened-in sleeping porches, and cross-ventilating windows be stressed in the design.

2. Make use of natural ventilation already present: throw open those windows. Do as they do in Italy—no screens—what flies in will find its way out. Once the sun hits the windows during the day, pull the blinds or close the curtains.

3. Use ceiling fans in every room. They're not only attractive, but functional; a cooling breeze during the summer can reduce your need for central air-conditioning. It also helps during the winter by circulating heat that gathers at the ceiling. Just use the reverse switch to change the direction of the fan blades. This will push the warm air down from the ceiling. A 2011 *New York Times* article by Michael Tortorello titled "Bringing in the Big Fans" offers extensive tips in this vein, as well as amusing tales of experimenting with alternate cooling methods.[36]

4. Use a whole-house fan. This fan, also known as an attic fan, provides ventilation, lowers indoor temperatures, and reduces electric bills. It pulls cooler outside air through open windows and sends hot indoor air out through the attic. It can lower the temperature in your home in just a few minutes. Another advantage of a whole-house fan is its cost—a few hundred dollars—compared to thousands of dollars for a central air conditioner.

5. Plant trees. Oaks, maples, and birches are all fast-growing trees that will shade your property for many years and will reduce temperatures beneath them. A complete tree résumé is available in a report from the University of Georgia. Prepare to be humbled: besides cutting heat, trees reduce carbon dioxide, wind, pollution, runoff, erosion, noise, glare, stress, and health care costs at the same time that they add value to a house sale and beauty to our lives.[37]

6. Choose correct clothing. Pick natural fabrics that breathe, such as silk, cotton, and linen. Avoid polyester and rayon. Performance fabrics, which wick heat away from the body, may be an exception to the synthetic ban. I learned this quickly while living in Egypt. People in desert cultures cover up from head to toe and not only for modesty; the loose light-colored cottons shade the skin from hot, harmful rays of the sun. The opposite holds true for dark colors. In Berlin—a city that forgets what sun looks like during gray winter months—light-absorbent black dominates the fashion scene.

Once inside your home or even someone else's, kick off those rubber sneakers or man-made soles. Heat naturally flees the body from the soles of the feet, the palms of the hands, and the top of our heads. Uncover them.

7. Eat the right foods. Certain foods will keep you cooler. Proteins lose some of their energy as heat—called the specific dynamic action of food—and as a result will make a person feel warmer. A steak dinner can keep the burn on for many hours. On the other hand, fruits and salads, low in fats and proteins but high in water content will keep body temperature down. Eat spicy food. It's not a coincidence that many people in hotter regions of the world eat spicy food. Curries from India and five-alarm Texan chili are good examples. Spicy food ratchets up sweat, which cools the body as it evaporates. Sweating is a good thing, not the bane deodorant ads would have you believe. Capsaicin, the fiery ingredient in chili peppers, is thought to promote weight loss by increasing fat oxidation.

8. *Become a more efficient heat dissipater.* When the weather starts heating up, resist the urge to turn on the air-conditioner. Sit outside on the porch or terrace, use a fan to circulate the air around your face, or have a Popsicle. Do some yoga. Try the downward-facing dog pose; panting is an effective heat dissipater. The body will take a few weeks to catch up to the change in temperature, but it will be much better at dispelling heat if it is allowed to experience some.

By replacing air-conditioning in your life with a bit more tolerance (acclimatization) and cooling techniques as outlined above, the calorie benefit will build over the years, and noticeably so over the decades. For example, a mere 25-calorie increase in energy expenditure coupled with 25 fewer calories eaten per day would prevent 5 extra pounds or so per year. No wonder we gain weight over a lifetime. We must change the approach. Calorie by calorie, thermostat by thermostat, and any other way we can fine-tune the energy equation of our metabolisms. Even a modest weight loss is important. Losing a few pounds reduces the risk for disease by lowering blood pressure and blood sugar and improving cholesterol levels. So, next summer when your family complains about how warm the house is, say you've turned down the air conditioner for health reasons. They might not like it at first but, as research shows, they will adapt. And maybe lose a few pounds as well.

2

. . . .

BACKSIDE EFFECTS:
DRUGS & OBESITY

Medications may cure what ails us, but some are
dangerously obesogenic.

CONSIDER THE FOLLOWING COMPLAINTS FROM consumers of a medication called Actos:

- *"Gained 50 pounds."* 54 year-old male on 30 mg Actos daily for 18 months. Posted April 3, 2012.

- *"Gained 20 pounds with no change in diet, I even tried to eat less and drink more water, and I was still gaining weight."* 42 year-old male on 15 mg Actos daily for 4 months. Posted November 26, 2011.

- *"I have never been overweight before. After 12 months of this drug, I have gained 50 lbs."* 50 year-old female on 15 mg Actos three times a day for 365 days. Posted October 10, 2011.

Many more on the popular website www.askapatient.com tell of crushing weight gain from the medication. The symptoms did not vary much; the fat came on fast and considerable for most posters.[1]

But here is the cruel irony: Actos is a standard drug prescribed to steady blood sugars in type 2 diabetes—a condition made worse by obesity. Weight gain will bring more of the same poor blood sugar control and thus need for more treatment.

This drug and too many others in modern pharmacies are pushing millions into the ranks of the overweight or obese. The same medications meant to keep disorders in check are likely to aggravate the problem or create a whole different set of troubles brought on by obesity. Surely biochemists would not choose this outcome for their disease-fighting formulas. Yet it is hard to ignore the fact that pharmaceutical companies benefit: overweight patients may continue to buy drugs for the rest of their lives.

While some scientists and clinicians may be aware of this unwelcome side effect, many patients first learn of it on the bathroom scale. The Internet is littered with tales of weight gain induced by drugs.

Five of the ten bestselling prescription drug classes in the United States in 2011 were linked to significant weight gain.[2] Chances are, you are taking at least one. Drugs for diabetes, depression, psychosis, high blood pressure, allergies, inflammation, and many others are guilty.

A broad review from the University of Glasgow linked many classes of drugs with weight gain, as much as 10 kilograms (kgs) or 22 pounds (lbs) in one year. In looking at 43 studies with 25,663 subjects, the authors found that "body weight and height are routinely recorded in virtually all clinical trials, but seldom reported."[3]

Evidently, research into the role of prescription drugs in weight gain is on the slim side. For obvious reasons, pharmaceutical companies are not keen on reporting that their pills will pile on the pounds. And why announce it when regulatory powers deem it a side effect of little import in the drug-approval process?

But weight gain does have consequences, very serious metabolic risks: raising blood sugars, blood pressures, and blood lipids, as well as trapping many in permanent inflammatory states. Adding to the problem is that so many people consume these obesogenic drugs on a chronic basis. Here's a troubling statistic from the Centers for Disease Control and Prevention (CDC): Among Americans over age 60, more than three-fourths take two or more prescription medications, and 37 percent of this age group used five or more.[4]

And as the enterprising pharmaceutical industry and its powerful marketing juggernaut assure more doctors and patients of the need for drugs, the rest of the world is catching up.

What's more, even if the drug treatment is mercifully short-term, the effects may be long lasting: once gained, weight is difficult to lose.

Is it a coincidence that obesity rates doubled in the last three decades as prescription drug use soared? Hardly. After reading the evidence in which so many medications add weight, you will see that simply choosing more carefully sounds like a potent plan for better health.

Much of the research is centered on US and UK populations. Statistics as well are hard to come by in many parts of the world. But the implications for global health are not good: prescription drug use is rising in tandem with obesity across the globe.

ANTIDIABETIC DRUGS

Diabetes is spreading faster than Nutella on warm cake.

Obesity and inactivity have bred record cases of new diabetics, both young and old, across the globe. In raw numbers, the problem is clear: in the United States, there are 25.8 million diabetics, according to data from a National Health Interview Survey.[5] Worldwide, about 285 million individuals are diabetic, with nearly a half billion predicted by 2030.[6]

Quick review: Type 2 diabetics—who in past decades had been called adult-onset until legions of children joined the ranks—become resistant to insulin, which they initially produce in normal amounts. Blood sugars stay high. These new cases differ from type 1 diabetes, an autoimmune disorder in which hormone-producing cells in the pancreas are destroyed leading to a scanty supply of insulin. In type 1 diabetes, insulin is given by injection or a pump.

Insulin replacement began in the 1920s; it must be given by injection because as a protein it would be digested passing through the stomach.

Yet most people prefer a pill to an injection.

It wasn't until World War II, when a French army doctor observed low blood sugars in soldiers on sulfa antibiotics, that oral meds to treat diabetes were introduced. It was a welcome breakthrough; needles were no longer needed.

For that reason, as well as an increase in diabetes and its

diagnosis, oral hypoglycemic use has skyrocketed. Adding to the number is a new role for the pills in a condition called pre-diabetes, which is a subtle state of glucose imbalance that predicts full-blown diabetes. The CDC reports that the use of antidiabetic drugs by American adults 45 years and over increased about 50 percent, from 7 percent in 1988–1994 to 11 percent in 2003–2006.[7]

Diabetes treatment is costly.

Insulin and glucose monitoring in type 1 are lifetime, unavoidable expenses. But type 2 diabetes can often be prevented or treated with lifestyle changes: diet, exercise, and weight loss. These cost nothing. The fourth leg of treatment is oral hypoglycemic drugs, a group that includes Actos. The American Diabetes Association estimated $245 billion was spent on diabetes care in 2012, a 41% jump from in 2007.[8] Marketing data in the United States show that prescriptions for oral antidiabetic agents increased from 23.3 million to 26.8 million between 2002 and 2006.[9]

Global spending on diabetes is expected to reach nearly a half trillion dollars by 2030, 12 percent of all health expenditures. In Nauru, that figure is already 41 percent of health care costs while in Saudi Arabia it is 21 percent.[10]

Rich nations have more diabetics than poor ones, a testament to pampered lifestyles. But as life modernizes for the even the poorest countries, their chronic health problems will grow.

Pharmaceutical companies formulate dozens of new medications to treat blood sugar problems. While most offer improvements, the business model also fills the drug pipeline as old drugs go off patent and face generic competitors; this means less profit than a branded drug.

The choice of one class of drug over another is obviously based on what works best for each patient. It is a difficult trial-by-error, one-size-definitely-doesn't-fit-all kind of business. Europeans may prefer one drug for diabetes whereas the United States might never have approved it. Marketing efforts and sales reach—and some will say the comeliness of the saleswomen—are also factors in which medication you are prescribed.

Each class has a unique way of lowering blood sugar. An antidiabetic drug may work by:

- Prompting the pancreas to make more insulin
- Improving the sensitivity of cells to insulin
- Blocking the action of stomach enzymes that break down carbohydrates
- Reducing the supply of glucose from the liver

Which Drugs for Diabetes Cause Weight Gain?

Sulfonylurea drugs were the first widely used oral hypoglycemic medications. They fuel insulin production. This in turn lowers blood sugar, an effect that may increase appetite.

In the United Kingdom Prospective Diabetes Study, a weight gain of 5.3 kilograms—nearly 12 pounds—with sulfonylureas was seen.[11] Studies comparing sulfonylureas to placebo[12] or another hypoglycemic agent[13] have shown weight increases of 1.4 kilograms (3.1 lbs.) to 2.3 kilograms (5.1 lbs.).[14]

Researchers at the University of Copenhagen in Denmark surveyed diabetics who were taking oral hypoglycemics about knowledge and worry regarding weight gain and hypoglycemia. A considerable number of patients with medications containing sulphonylurea were not even aware of these possible side effects.[15]

Thiazolidinediones, also called glitazones, are the newer kids on the prescription pad. Actos is in this group. Introduced in the late 1990s, this class boosts insulin sensitivity; cells accept more glucose, which removes sugar from blood but can end up storing it as fat.

Rosiglitazone and pioglitazone are top sellers. Both have come under scrutiny (as was another called troglitazone, which was retired because of harm to the liver), the first for heart risks and the latter for bladder cancer links.

Still this group remains very popular. Prescriptions climbed from 7.8 million in 2002 to 12.6 million in 2006 in the United States. In just four years, sales went up over 60 percent. Global markets were similar.[16]

So why do people gain weight with these particular drugs? One big reason is that less glucose is lost in the urine because insulin is ferrying it into cells; as a result, patients consume more calories to fight dips in blood sugar and then extra energy is stored as fat. And thiazolidinediones spur appetite by decreasing leptin. Fluid retention is another common cause of weight gain in this class. And yet another way, said researcher Rosane Ness-Abramof of Tel Aviv University in Israel is that glitazones have a direct effect on differentiation of adipocytes. In other words, more fat cells are made.

OTHER ANTIDIABETIC DRUGS

Biguanides are derived from *Galega officinalis*, a lilac plant used in folk medicine for several centuries. They hinder release of glucose from liver and improve sensitivity to insulin. Also, they can reduce LDL cholesterol, another substantial perk in the health department. Biguanides seem to have no effect on weight or possibly even lead to decrease in weight.[17]

One of these called metformin appears to be safe and effective.[18] It improves blood sugar control at a lower price than many other oral hypoglycemics and doesn't cause weight gain. In the United Kingdom Prospective Diabetes Study mentioned earlier, a weight gain of 5.3 kilograms (11.68 lbs.) was seen with sulfonylureas but a weight loss of 1.3 kilograms (2.87 lbs.) with metformin.

Metformin is now believed to be the most widely prescribed antidiabetic drug in the world. Metformin does sound like a miracle drug. So why are people still taking pills that cause weight gain? And why did it take so long to be accepted in the United States by the FDA? Metformin was introduced to the United Kingdom in 1958, Canada in 1972, and only became available in the United States in 1995.

For one, metformin isn't perfect. It can lend a metallic taste to food and can cause gut upset—two side effects that are undesirable but at the same time will reduce food intake. More dangerous are the risks to liver and kidneys. People with already compromised organs or heavy drinkers may be advised to avoid metformin. And metformin doesn't appear to work as well in some cases, such as in preventing people with impaired glucose tolerance from converting to diabetes. The gliazides work better for this. In one study, pioglitazone decreased the risk of conversion to diabetes by 72 percent.

But "the mean weight gain in patients treated with pioglitazone was 3.6 kilograms" (7.93 lbs.). However, in a puzzling twist, "the greater the weight gain, the greater the improvements in beta-cell function and insulin sensitivity, and thus the greater the reduction in HbA_{1c}."[19] Metformin reduced the development of type 2 diabetes by 31 percent in the U.S. Diabetes Prevention Program.[20]

One more explanation may be this: People prescribed weight-gainers may likely stay on them. "Why rock the boat?" is a philosophy with multiple medication therapies. Unless the patient complains, the first drugs stay put. People stay on the same medications for years even as weight changes and metabolic markers improve. This clinical inertia is not ideal for health. Is the diabetes drug keeping the HbA_{1c} in good stead or something else? A short stint with a lesser dose or even without the drug may be something you and your doctor should consider together.

There are other types of drugs to lower glucose that don't add weight though they may have other side effects. One called *alpha-glucosidase inhibitor* works by preventing enzymes in the gut from digesting carbohydrates. This keeps the sugar out of the bloodstream but can cause flatulence. The good news is they don't impact weight. Acarbose or Precose are examples.

Newer treatments named *incretin mimetics* and *DPP-4 inhibitors* provide good control of both blood sugar and body weight. Traditional treatments for type 2 diabetes have focused on impaired insulin secretion and insulin resistance but these new ones attack the underlying dysfunction.

Some type 2 diabetics eventually require insulin, which can also add weight. One study found that people gained nearly 11 pounds on average during their first three years taking insulin. But certain types of insulin, such as long-acting insulin, have less extreme effects.

Diabetes threatens not only health but the financial stability of families and entire countries. Insulin and pills are only a tip of deeper medical problems: blindness, amputations, kidney failure, and other complications of diabetes will engulf budgets. People with diabetes require at least two to three times the resources compared to people without diabetes. Moreover, diabetes care can take as much as one-third of income in poor countries.

SOLUTIONS

Prevention of type 2 diabetes is key. It can be done. But people must change how they eat and move more. As many as 13 percent of those with impaired glucose tolerance cross over each year to full-blown diabetes.[21]

The Diabetes Prevention Study (DPS) and the Diabetes Prevention Program (DPP) showed that lifestyle changes could reduce the risk of diabetes by as much as 58 percent[22] and even more in older adults.[23]

- Increase in dietary fiber (≥15 g/1000 kcal)
- Reduction of total fat (< 30% of energy consumed)
- Reduction of saturated fat (< 10% of energy consumed)
- Moderate physical activity (≥30 min/day)

Most adults with diabetes are obese.[24] The American Diabetes Association (ADA) has published a joint statement with the North American Association for the Study of Obesity and the American Society for Clinical Nutrition recommending a moderate weight loss (5 percent of body weight) to "improve insulin action, decrease fasting blood glucose level, and reduce the need for anti-diabetes medications."[25] That is only 10 pounds in a person weighing 200 pounds.

Still, weight loss is difficult to maintain. And nearly half of individuals with impaired glucose tolerance will progress to type 2 diabetes over their lifetimes despite successful weight reduction. For these people, medications will be needed. Different patients will need different regimens based on their genetic and cultural backgrounds as well as other medical problems. But physicians should aim first for blood sugar control with drugs or a combination of drugs that don't spur weight gain.

One radical solution shows promise. Studies showed that bariatric surgery (banding or cutting parts of the gastrointestinal tract) in morbidly obese subjects sent about three out of four with type 2 diabetes into remission following the procedure. The drastic drop in food consumption along with metabolic changes is thought to drive the rapid improvement, within days of surgery in some cases, in blood sugar control.[26]

ANTIDEPRESSANTS

In 2011 antidepressants beat out lipid regulators to become the most dispensed drug in America. The number of prescriptions written that year reached an unprecedented 264 million.[27]

Were we always this unhappy?

No doubt but now pills make sure we don't stay that way. Prozac and its offspring Lexapro, Zoloft, Cymbalta, and Abilify have lifted spirits faster than a sunny day in Seattle. Spending on just one drug used in depression, aripiprazole, more than doubled in the last five years.[28] The United Kingdom, France, and Australia also reported large jumps in antidepressant drug usage in the past two decades.[29]

People love them.

Unfortunately, weight gain is one of the most common side effects for most antidepressants. The obesity epidemic may be partially explained by the widespread use of these drugs. Some are worse than others. One group called the tricyclic antidepressants has been recognized for years as a cause of weight gain. Several studies show that weight gain ranged from one to three pounds per month during treatment with tricyclic antidepressants. Specific tricyclics that have been associated with weight gain include nortriptyline, doxepin, and amitriptyline.[30]

The last one in that trio has been around for over 40 years and is linked to considerable weight gain.[31] Amitriptyline treats more than a few problems: in addition to depression, it is prescribed for anxiety, attention deficit, migraines, eating disorders, bipolar disorder, insomnia, and post-herpetic neuralgia, but also provides relief for chronic pain, tinnitus, carpal tunnel syndrome, fibromyalgia, vulvodynia, interstitial cystitis, male chronic pelvic pain syndrome, irritable bowel syndrome, laryngeal sensory neuropathy, chronic fatigue syndrome, and multiple sclerosis.

Waistlines have widened right along with its job description.

What causes this weight gain? Scientists suspect that mood improvement makes people eat more. So weight gain may be one sign they are working. And if the disease caused weight loss, then recovery may mean weight gain.

Another cause may be changes in brain chemistry. The tricyclics affect neurotransmitters involved in managing energy and appetite, such as serotonin, dopamine, and acetylcholine. And a 2011 study from Italy suggests neuropeptide changes to be the problem.[32]

They also exert antihistamine activity, which some think is the weight gain mechanism.

Not every antidepressant is at fault. Selective serotonin reuptake inhibitors (SSRIs) don't usually cause weight gain because the serotonin surge increases satiety, not hunger. But there are exceptions. Researchers at Massachusetts General Hospital in Boston looked at weight changes in patients randomly assigned to treatment with fluoxetine, sertraline, or paroxetine.

More patients treated with paroxetine than with either fluoxetine or sertraline gained at least 7 percent of original weight during 26 to 32 weeks of treatment.[33] Even so, drugs which don't trigger weight gain initially can do so later.[34]

"Antidepressants such as amitriptyline, mirtazapine, and some serotonin reuptake inhibitors (SSRIs) [may cause] weight gain that cannot be explained solely by improvement in [depression]. The same phenomenon is observed with mood stabilizers such as lithium, valproic acid, and carbamazepine," according to review from researchers at Tel Aviv University in Israel.[35]

Some of the newer antidepressants may be less fattening. A class called atypical appears not to cause an uptick in pounds. One of these called nefazodone is weight neutral[36] and a second, bupropion, may induce weight loss.[37]

Another worry is the hit-or-miss nature of treatment. Patients try one drug after another until the right alchemy makes them feel better. Often a cocktail of different drugs is prescribed, which multiplies harmful side effects, including weight gain. Furthermore, after decades of explosive growth in use, the low-serotonin theory of depression is being challenged across scientific disciplines.[38] Could patients feel just as good with a sugar pill?

Many patients do abandon the drugs after a short run because of side effects. But the effects of the drug may linger long after you stopped taking them. In one recent experiment, rats were exposed to stress and short-term antidepressant treatment. Then the drug was stopped, but the animals had access to a high-fat chow. Guess what? Even after the drug was stopped, they gained more weight than their rodent dining partners who had never had antidepressants.[39]

This is discouraging news in light of the obesity epidemic. Antidepressants can continue to cause weight gain even after treatment is finished.

Moreover, weight gain is not considered a serious side effect by many clinicians. On drugs.com, an information site, patients who are prescribed one antidepressant are told to tell their doctor about serious side effects such as headaches but not for a "less serious side effect" of weight gain. Many clinical trials don't even include weight changes in their data—an odd omission given the fact that many people are already overweight.

Ideas for management of weight gain caused by the use of antidepressants follow the next section on psychotropic drugs.

ANTIPSYCHOTICS

Moving deeper into the mind meld are psychotropic drugs. These drugs are prescribed for schizophrenia, psychosis, borderline personality, mania, alcohol dependence, and bipolar disorders, as well as a few others.

Psychotropic drug use is soaring. Usage in the US climbed from 6.1 percent to 11.1 percent of the population between the period of the third NHANES from 1988–1994 and NHANES 1999–2002.[40] And according to the IMS Institute for Healthcare Informatics, people in America filled 57 million prescriptions in 2011, up nearly 70 percent since 2002.[41] The explosion in use of antipsychotic drugs was reported by Robert Whitaker in his chilling 2010 book *Anatomy of an Epidemic*.[42] As many as one in five Americans takes a psychiatric drug regularly, according to recent industry data from Medco Health Solutions.[43] Whitaker's contention was that with so many on these drugs, mental illness should be subsiding. Instead his investigation found that the drugs may be making them worse, not only mentally but also physically, from liver damage, diabetes, and obesity. The vast number of prescriptions being written for these drugs is a force behind the obesity epidemic.

Let's begin with a brief glimpse into the world of psychotropic drugs.

Thorazine (chlorpromazine) was the first major antipsychotic. Introduced nearly 60 years ago, Thorazine was associated with weight gain even then. New generations of more effective drugs followed: olanzapine, risperidone, and quetiapine in the 1990s; ziprasidone and aripiprazole in the early 2000s; and approved by the FDA in late 2006, the atypical antipsychotic paliperidone. Atypicals are popular because they limit certain side effects including extrapyramidal symptoms.

But weight gain, unfortunately, persists. Antipsychotics, with rare exception, put weight on, often enough to take the patient from normal weight to overweight or obese. Some will have minor effect while others are disastrous for the scales.[44] Antipsychotics are also equal opportunity thickeners: weight gain occurs no matter what the patient's age, race, or gender.

Clozapine and olanzipine are the most fattening. These drugs are used for schizophrenia and bipolar disorders.

A meta-analysis conducted in Birmingham, United Kingdom, revealed that patients treated with clozapine and olanzapine have higher rates of weight gain and more type 2 diabetes compared to those on other antipsychotics.[45]

An earlier review of 81 articles reported a weight gain of 4.45 kilograms (9.81 lbs.) for clozapine and 4.15 kilograms (9.15 lbs.) for olanzapine after only 10 weeks.[46] And remember these drugs are taken for long periods, if not a lifetime. Weight continued to mount with clozapine treatment for as long as 46 months in one study.[47] And get this: diabetic symptoms surfaced faster than could be predicted by weight gain alone. In fact, glucose and lipids are quickly disrupted by the drug, even before the pounds accumulate.[48]

One trial looked at patients assigned to olanzapine for a first-episode psychosis. After two years, the mean weight gain was 15.4 kilograms or about 34 pounds. Virtually all of the patients were predicted to gain more than 7 percent of their initial body weight after one year of treatment.[49]

With few exceptions (ziprasidone and molindone), all of the newer agents are associated with significantly greater weight gain than placebo.

How Does This Happen?

Appetite surges. Interestingly, male rats responded differently than females: males had less weight gain and didn't eat as much on the drug. Human females are far more likely to binge eat than males. One study found that 22.2 percent of the female patients and 6.4 percent of the males binged when both clozapine and olanzapine were taken together.[50]

Calorie intake goes up.[51] This may be partly explained by hormones. Blood levels of the appetite hormone leptin doubled during the first two weeks of treatment in eight of twelve study patients at the Department of Child and Adolescent Psychiatry of the University of Marburg, Germany. Low doses of clozapine were enough to induce this effect. Weight, BMI, fat mass, and lean body mass all increased within a ten-week period.[52]

Changes in the brain may also account for appetite response. A study at the University of Montreal was designed to examine changes in the brain activity associated with 16 weeks of olanzapine treatment in schizophrenic patients. Nineteen men and five women were recruited for the study.[53] Researchers reported, "After 16 weeks of olanzapine treatment, the patients gained weight, increased waist circumference, had fewer positive schizophrenia symptoms, a reduced ghrelin plasma concentration, and an increased concentration of triglycerides, insulin and leptin." In addition, all of the participants underwent MRIs while they looked at either neutral images (a rock, hammer, and so on) or appetizing ones (cake, pizza, and so on). Brain activity jumped in the schizophrenic patients as they viewed foods, notably in the part that is assigned appetite duty. These changes also correlated to the changes in insulin, leptin, and ghrelin. Schizophrenics were more sensitive to external cues in their decisions to eat.

With animal studies, researchers observed that olanzapine increased fat deposits by four distinct routes: decreased physical activity, more glucose going into fat tissue, more fatty acids going into fat tissue, and, finally, fat becoming trapped.[54]

Another suspect is the antihistamine activity of the drugs; sleepiness and inactivity lower energy expenditure.

We are willing to put up with side effects of drugs in many medical conditions. The collateral damage ranges from the merely annoying such as dry mouth from antiallergenics to the almost lethal in cancer treatments. But weight gain, though insidious, should also be feared; once gained, it is hard to remove and proceeds to chip away at health and can shorten lives, especially in people with chronic mental health illnesses.

A team of researchers in Pakistan were concerned about weight gain in their psychiatric patients. They reviewed the records of those who had been prescribed antipsychotic medication at the psychiatry outpatient clinic of Aga Khan University Hospital in Karachi, Pakistan, over a four-year period.[55]

Though half of the patients were already overweight, more weight followed when the drugs started. On average, patients gained about 2 kilograms (4.41 lbs.) and 3.5 kilograms (7.72 lbs.) in 3 and 6 months, respectively. This correlated with BMI increases. It is interesting that Pakistan and other Asian populations abide by lower BMI cutoff points to determine overweight and obesity. The World Health Organization (WHO) consultation suggested the intervals of < 18.5, 18.5 to 23, 23 to 27.5 and ≥ 27.5, representing the categories of being underweight, increasing but acceptable risk, increased risk, and higher risk, respectively.[56]

Which drugs brought on the most weight gain for the Pakistanis? On olanzapine, 71 percent gained, whereas 51 percent did on risperidone, and 16 percent on quetiapine. Pakistanis may have an increased risk for using these drugs because diabetes rates are much higher than Western countries. They also reported that "the overall prevalence of diabetes mellitus in Pakistan has been reported to be between 8.6 percent and 13.9 percent." Any drug that causes weight gain is, therefore, likely to have even more serious consequences in terms of morbidity and mortality for the Pakistani population.[57]

Weight gain may be considered by many clinicians and patients alike to be a small price to pay for peace of mind. The problem is that weight gain, especially in the numbers we have seen, leads to different problems in the guise of diabetes and heart disease, which lead to pain and early death. Because schizophrenics are already prone to poor health, obesity only exacerbates it. Mental health suffers too as many patients may decide not to take their meds because of this unappealing side effect. Fortunately, there may be alternatives.

SOLUTIONS

1. Doctors should consider switching

Given the risks to health and treatment compliance associated with weight gain and obesity, clinicians should monitor weight during the course of antipsychotic therapy and consider switching agents if excessive weight gain occurs. Often alternative medications can be prescribed. If no acceptable alternatives exist, the minimal dosage should be tried.[58, 59, 60]

Switching to weight-neutral antipsychotics like ziprasidone and aripiprazole may cause less weight gain.

2. Dietary counseling should be part of every prescription.

Authors of the research in Pakistan concluded that "it is important that while initiating an antipsychotic medication in this patient population, psychiatrists should counsel patients about the risk of weight gain associated with antipsychotic use, the increased risk of morbidity and mortality associated with weight gain, and the lifestyle changes such as changes in dietary habits and regular exercise that the patients can adopt to counter that risk." Weight management advice and programs should start with every drug. The interaction will also be helpful. Unfortunately, many insurance companies only pay for dietary counseling for diabetes or coinciding with bariatric surgery. A healthy diet is the cornerstone of health and registered dietitians can guide us. The Academy of Nutrition and Dietetics can locate a registered dietitian near you. Go to www.EatRight.org.

3. Exercise is crucial.

Physical activity increases mental health. A researcher at Charite hospital in Berlin, Germany, looked at the literature regarding exercise and its effect on psychiatric disorders. Exercise was found to be effective in major depression and panic disorder.[61] And a 2011 review from the Medical University of South Carolina cites several studies supporting the use of exercise as a treatment for depression. The researchers concluded that "exercise compares favorably to anti-depressant medications as a first-line treatment for mild to moderate depression and has also been shown to improve depressive symptoms when used as an adjunct to medications. While not as extensively studied, exercise has been shown to be an effective and cost-efficient treatment alternative for a variety of anxiety disorders." Inactivity, they noted, was linked with the development of psychological disorders.[62]

Our species was not bred to sit at computers and televisions all day.

A group of researchers from Belgium took this several steps further. They wondered how intensity, type of activity, duration, and frequency would impact different types of mental disorders. Their subjects were in-patients at the hospital. The 128 men were mostly suffering from major depressive disorder, anxiety disorders, and alcoholism. The depressed patients showed the most interest in exercise. Improvement was clear in those who exercised with cycling and gymnastics offering the most benefit.[63]

4. Some other ideas

St. John's wort, or *Hypericum perforatum*, is commonly used in Germany for depression. The herb did better than both placebo and antidepressants in trials conducted in Europe. When it was used in a blinded trial in the United States, St. John's wort performed about the same as Zoloft but neither did as well as a placebo.[64] "Recent . . . studies suggest that St. John's wort is involved in the regulation of genes that control hypothalamic-pituitary-adrenal axis function."[65] It doesn't cause weight gain. It is available as a supplement.

Omega-3 fatty acids. These are found in cold-water fish, flaxseed, flax oil, walnuts, and some other foods. Eating a diet rich in omega-3s or taking omega-3 supplements may help ease depression.

Folate. This may be helpful when used in addition to antidepressants. Ask a dietitian what amount is right for you.

Other techniques that may be tried to ease depression and mental disorders include acupuncture, yoga, meditation, guided imagery, massage, and cognitive therapy.

ANTIEPILEPTICS

Valproic acid is used to treat bipolar disorder and seizures as well as to prevent migraines. A 2007 study of epilepsy patients found that 44 percent of women and 24 percent of men gained 11 pounds or more while taking valproic acid for about a year. [66] The drug affects proteins involved in appetite and metabolism, although it's not clear why it appears to affect women more than men. According to another study in 2005, "Antiepileptic drugs that promote weight gain include valproate, carbamazepine, and gabapentin. Lamotrigine is . . . weight-neutral, while topiramate and zonisamide may induce weight loss.[67]

Lithium for bipolar disease has been used for four decades. Weight gain reported is substantial, up to 35 pounds in some cases.[68]

SOLUTIONS

These patients should be carefully monitored after drug therapy begins. Physicians should advise the patient on potential weight changes and refer to a dietitian when needed.

HIGH BLOOD PRESSURE DRUGS

As many as a billion people on the planet struggle with high blood pressure, putting all at risk of stroke, heart attack, and early death. It wasn't always this way. Obesity, aging populations, and poor diets have not made it easy on our magnificent river under the skin.

Pharmaceutical companies have come up with a Damien Hirst-like selection to bring the numbers down. The many medicines used to treat high blood pressure include

- Alpha-blockers
- Angiotensin-converting enzyme (ACE) inhibitors
- Angiotensin receptor blockers (ARBs)
- Beta-blockers
- Calcium channel blockers

- Central alpha agonists

- Diuretics

- Renin inhibitors

- Vasodilators

As is often the case, finding the best is a gamble of trial and error. Frequently, two or more are combined for a hypertension cocktail.

Beta-blockers are often included. These drugs are well known to add weight: atenolol, metoprolol, and propranolol. A look at beta-blockers against control groups revealed a median weight gain difference of 1.2 kilograms or nearly three pounds for the first group.[69]

Why?

It could be that beta-blockers slow your metabolism.[70]

Also, if you switch from taking a diuretic to a beta-blocker as treatment for high blood pressure, you may gain a few pounds of water weight that the diuretic had kept off. Weight gain may mean something ominous in the short term: fluid retention in the legs or chest, which signals heart trouble.

Thus in their small way, some antihypertensive drugs contribute to the obesity epidemic.

SOLUTIONS

1. Doctors should consider a switch

There are alternatives to avoid weight gain. The best solution may also be the cheapest: a simple diuretic created nearly 60 years ago. And there are newer beta-blockers that don't cause weight gain.

To find a better way, look to the causes: poor diet and inactivity. Experts agree that lifestyle changes could lower most pressures just as well as any pill.[71]

2. Diet

If you feel you know everything about this part, think again. While low salt restrictions anchor the advice, new functional foods and nutrients also help.

Follow the DASH (Dietary Approaches to Stop Hypertension) diet.

The DASH diet's eating plan is rich in fruits, vegetables, whole grains, fish, poultry, nuts and legumes, and low-fat dairy. These foods are high in key nutrients such as potassium, magnesium, calcium, fiber, and protein.

- Grains: 7–8 daily servings
- Vegetables: 4–5 daily servings
- Fruits: 4–5 daily servings
- Low-fat or fat-free dairy products: 2–3 daily servings
- Lean meat, poultry, and fish: 2 or fewer servings a day
- Nuts, seeds, and legumes: 4–5 servings per week
- Fats and oils: 2–3 daily servings
- Sweets: limit to fewer than 5 servings per week.

Aim to cut back to 2,300 milligrams of sodium per day (about one teaspoon of table salt). Once your body adjusts to the lower-sodium diet, you can lower your salt intake even further to 1,500 milligrams per day (about ⅔ teaspoon table salt). As many as half of those with hypertension are sensitive to salt. This means that a lower salt intake will result in lower blood pressure.

Probiotics figure in blood pressure control. These microbes act on a milk protein called casein, churning out peptides that act as angiotensin I-converting enzyme (ACE) inhibitors. Sound familiar? ACE is the key enzyme in the rennin-angiotensin system and plays an important role in regulating blood pressure. Medications known as ACE inhibitors are prescribed for this action.

Functional foods also show promise: These include L-arginine, garlic, onion, tea, soybean, ginger, hawthorn, and fish oil.[72]

3. Exercise

Physical activity is the cornerstone for prevention and control of high blood pressure. The best? Endurance exercise such as walks and bicycle rides can prevent and lower blood pressure. Studies show that blood pressure is reduced for up to 22 hours after this type of exercise. How much and how often to do any good? That answer seems to change weekly but the American College of Sports Medicine position advises at least 30 minutes every day. Supplement with resistance training.[73]

Researchers at Tulane University combed 54 different studies and found that aerobic exercise reduced blood pressure significantly.[74]

And not surprisingly, yoga, with its numerous stress-relieving benefits, also brings the numbers down in hypertension.[75]

ANTIRETROVIRAL THERAPY AND PROTEASE INHIBITORS

Skeletal images of human immunodeficiency disease (HIV) victims are tragic. Seeing weight gain from the new antiretroviral therapies would be a certain relief. However, as HIV now requires chronic treatment over a lifetime, weight increase may be troublesome if it leads to obesity and all its risks.

These drugs tend to add fat in the abdominal area. One study of 10 HIV patients given protease inhibitors found a 19-pound average weight gain after just six months.[76]

A more recent study from Children's Hospital of Philadelphia looked at the impact of antiretroviral therapy on children with HIV. The authors concluded that while "antiretroviral therapy improves survival and growth in children with HIV infection," it is linked to "adverse changes in body composition and metabolism." Under the umbrella called lipodystrophy, children on the therapy can experience insulin resistance, dyslipidemia, and relocation of fat tissue. Children with HIV are at greater risk due to a potential lifetime exposure to the drugs.[77]

SOLUTIONS

Researchers in Brazil advise health-care workers to encourage HIV patients to change lifestyle and unhealthy social habits, choose individual antiretroviral regimens that combine the least toxic with greater antiviral activity, and decide if a lipid-lowering agent is needed.[78]

GASTROESOPHAGEAL REFLUX DISEASE DRUGS (GERD)

This very common condition was formerly known as heartburn. Typical symptoms of acid regurgitation and burn can lead to esophagitis and other complications. In the old days, a baking soda cocktail or a handful of Tums were the few remedies available to buffer stomach acid. Other changes thought to bring relief by reducing acid or at least by discouraging its stinging backwash were elevation of the head of the bed; decreased intake of fat, chocolate, alcohol, peppermint, coffee, onions, and garlic; cessation of smoking; and avoiding lying down for three hours after eating. Weight loss also helped.

Still, because people continued to smoke, drink, and of course, eat, a pharmaceutical remedy was sought. Proton-pump inhibitors (PPIs) fit the bill. They work fast and have become the heart of GERD treatment.

Losing weight once was the first-line therapy for GERD but no longer; PPIs are easier and readily available. And highly profitable for their makers. PPIs comprise the largest outpatient pharmacy expenditure in the United States.

Here's the problem: The cure can induce weight gain, which in turn causes more reflux, which then requires more of the cure. This vicious cycle is beneficial for the drug companies but less positive for the millions with reflux.

Researchers in Japan evaluated 52 adult patients with GERD and 58 healthy controls. GERD patients were treated with PPI for a mean of 2.2 years; average weight increase in 37 patients was 3.5 kilograms (7.72 lbs.). Most of the control group (91%) remained stable, within a 5 percent change, compared to weight at the baseline.[79]

This study demonstrated that long-term PPI treatment is linked with undesirable body weight gain in patients with GERD.

How does this happen?

First, people eat more when they aren't in pain. PPIs relieve the pain, calorie intake goes up, more weight follows, and GERD can become chronic. Even a small weight gain among normal weight persons results in development or exacerbation of symptoms in GERD patients.[80]

And not surprisingly, stomach acid has purpose and it's not to irritate us. Its duties include breaking down food and absorbing nutrients, two tasks known to most people. But it is also essential for pancreas and gallbladder function as well as microbial health. Energy balance depends on each of these.

SOLUTIONS

Go back to square one. Try to lose weight first; you may prevent GERD altogether or at least reduce the duration or dosage of PPIs. And give your body time to improve. Use the advice old-timers espouse, such as elevating the head of the bed and other suggestions listed a few pages ago. Often it will resolve itself.

ASTHMA MEDICATIONS

The epidemic of asthma points to environmental toxins; its treatment leads to obesity.

Hydrocortisone, prednisone, and cortisone are chemically similar to the hormones made in the adrenal glands. The side effects of these drugs are well documented: weight distribution to the back of the neck, face, and abdomen; fluid retention; and general weight gain pose additional problems.

Oral corticosteroids, such as prednisone, are more potent than inhaled forms and carry a higher risk of weight gain, particularly with long-term use.

One study showed a 2.0 kilograms (4.41 lbs.) weight gain after 24 weeks in patients taking prednisone.[81]

A 2006 survey of long-term oral-corticosteroid users suggested that 60 to 80 percent had gained weight.

SOLUTIONS

It can be hard to counteract the side effects of long-term steroid use, but patients can be warned of possible weight gain so as to adjust physical activity and diet.

ORAL CONTRACEPTIVES

Name the one invention that changed more in the twentieth century than anything else? Probably "the Pill." So famous it can go by one name, like Cher and Madonna, the birth control pill forever changed the balance of power between men and women. Does it make women heavier too?

Many women on the pill say yes, but there is little to back it up.

In 2011, the CDC scoured many databases for research in this vein. They found 49 trials to examine. No evidence linking combination oral contraceptives or a combination skin patch and weight change was seen.[82]

Nevertheless many clinicians and women believe an association exists.

One study of Navajo women in Albuquerque, New Mexico, indicated an average excess weight gain of six pounds at one year and eleven pounds at two years on Depo-medroxyprogesterone acetate. Native American women have extremely high rates of obesity and future study may find that birth control pills are one cause.[83]

Meanwhile, the problem here is that many women discontinue contraception and face unwanted pregnancies if they believe they are gaining weight, which in some cases may be bloating from fluid retention or even just natural tendencies to gain weight with aging. Physicians and clinicians should discuss alternate means of contraception—IUDs, barrier methods, and others as well as relative success rates with them.

ALLERGY DRUGS

Antihistamine users also report weight gain. It is thought that the stronger the antihistamine, the greater the potential for weight gain.[84] Often this class of drug causes sleepiness. A drop in exercise can follow. In addition, insulin levels are altered with these drugs, which may contribute to obesity.[85]

SOLUTIONS

Probiotics can often alleviate allergic reactions, thus reducing your need for antihistamine drugs. Get plenty of fermented foods including yogurt, kefir, and kimchee in your diet.

PULLING IT ALL TOGETHER

Prescription and over-the-counter drug use continues to soar across the globe. Half of the bestsellers can cause weight gain, shocking amounts in some cases. Oral hypoglycemics for diabetes, beta-blockers for high blood pressure, tricyclics for depression, proton pump inhibitors for acid reflux . . . all of these can interfere with normal metabolism or appetite control. Ironically, these added pounds perpetuate the very disorders the medications are targeting.

Of course, many pharmaceuticals are vital to control diseases and dangerous outcomes. Lives are saved. Thus weight gain should not stop usage. For these people, extra help through referral to a dietitian should be given to manage weight. The underlying causes of the problem should be treated as well. Yet too many prescriptions are written without regard for their metabolic mischief. A more cynical person may even view this guaranteed pipeline for future sales as less than coincidental.

The answer is not to refuse meds, but for more action on everyone's part: We as consumers should practice good defense by learning about side effects as well as alternative methods of preventing and treating diseases. Doctors should track weight in patients and give gains as well as losses the attention they deserve. Drug companies should record and publish weight changes.

First do no harm—it's a credo the health care industry should revisit.

3

. . . .

PRICE OF EFFLUENCE: POLLUTION & OBESITY

Pollution from air, water, and too many other sources gets under our skin and more, causing changes that lead to obesity.

POLLUTION CAUSES OBESITY. STRONG CHARGE— and some may say a convenient excuse for big appetites and little exercise—but solid evidence proves the case. From Riyadh to Cairo to London to Los Angeles to Jakarta to Beijing and most places in between, bad stuff in our air, food, and water is trashing our physiques.

These twin evils, pollution and obesity, are no strangers. As obesity rates have exploded in the last half century, chemicals have dramatically changed the environment.

"It is plausible and provocative to associate the recent increased incidence of obesity with a rapid increase in the use of industrial chemicals over the past 40 [years]," wrote researchers Felix Grün and Bruce Blumberg in a 2006 issue of *Endocrinology*.[1]

Many of these chemicals cause weight gain. In fact, some were designed for that purpose: growth hormones to fatten livestock and drugs to add pounds in malnourished patients. But most—bisphenol A (BPA) in your baby's bottle, pesticides on your lawn, and the nonstick finish in your frying pan as well as hundreds of others—are unintentionally altering our bodies and making us fat.

Indeed, research reveals, "the current level of human exposure to these chemicals may have damaged many of the body's natural weight-control mechanisms. . . . These effects together with a wide range of additional, possibly synergistic, factors may play a significant role in the worldwide obesity epidemic."[2]

Wow, how do people begin to assess the level of pollution and toxic exposure in their lives? Cairo, where I live, has some of the dirtiest air and water in the world. On a rare clear day, you can see the pyramids from miles away but, on most days, only the nearby Sphinx and tourists can vouch for their existence. In Cairo, air quality is dinner conversation and surgical masks are not confined to hospitals. No one is swimming in the Nile.

I do know this: if you live in a city where companies pay employees extra for the hit to their health, you're in deep trouble.

Never lived in a big polluted city? Unfortunately, you're not out of danger. Even if your small town boasts of clean air and pristine water, harmful chemicals still lurk in other places. Some, such as lawn pesticides, oven cleaner, and insect spray, are not a surprise. The fumes alone betray the poison inside the can. But suspicion is now cast on a wider tangle of chemicals: the flame retardant in your child's pajamas, the resin cemented in your teeth, the plastic in your baby's bottle, the whitening agent in your toothpaste, the special ingredient in your moisturizer, the filter in your sunscreen, the antimicrobial in your soap, the paraffin in your candle, the formaldehyde in your bookshelf, and the list goes on. And worse, we haven't even gotten to the kitchen, where many additional harmful chemicals infest food. Upon hearing this, many may wonder, "Why don't I have cancer?" instead of "Why me?" In addition to cancer, many of these are known to fuel emphysema, asthma, and heart disease. And now obesity.

A role for pollutants in the obesity epidemic is more recent, but every bit as distressing.

In 2002, researcher Paula Baillie-Hamilton of Scotland published a seminal paper that stated that the current obesity epidemic could not be explained solely by poor diet and inactivity. She wrote: "What has, up to now, been overlooked is that the earth's environment has changed significantly during the last few decades because of the exponential production and usage of synthetic organic and inorganic chemicals."[3]

She then named many studies in which chemicals spurred weight gain. The list included more familiar ones like phthalates, bisphenol A (BPA), and pesticides but also others not known to many outside of a lab.

How was this happening? Baillie-Hamilton thought the chemicals were changing hormones, neurotransmitters, or the sympathetic nervous system. "Many of these chemicals are better known for causing weight loss at high levels of exposure, but much lower concentrations of these same chemicals have powerful weight-promoting actions," she reported.

More recently, Retha Newbold of the National Institute of Environmental Health Sciences, part of the National Institutes of Health, added to the alarm. Her charge? Exposure to environmental chemicals during development—before birth—may be contributing to the obesity epidemic.[4]

The case is building: common chemicals can make us fat.

Because there are so many, toxins are classified in public health circles by source of exposure. If the periodic table makes you weep, know that you are not alone. Nevertheless, it is crucial to learn what sort of chemical soup our industrial giants are serving to us and, as it turns out, to generations far in the future.

Environmental Nutrition, a textbook written by registered dietitian Buck Levin, is a good place to start; he does an excellent job of explaining the difficult language of toxins.[5] For our purpose of linking to obesity, the threats will be addressed in the following order: indoor air, innermost air (the womb), outdoor air, and, finally, water.

INDOOR AIR

Berlin, Germany, devotes one-third of its city to forests, lakes, beaches, and other natural spaces. When I lived there, I would bike in a designated lane for many hours through local woods called the Grunewald; in fact, one can ride nearly uninterrupted to Sweden. The air was fresh and clean and felt healthy in Berlin. Indoors was another matter. Smokers everywhere. Candles and paraffin fumes lighting the gray winters. Mold growing in dank ceilings.

Indoor air pollution takes many forms, wherever on the planet you call home or office. Air quality, writes Levin, can be compromised by smoke, poor ventilation, presence of pollens and molds, presence of microorganisms, release of chemical fumes and gases, faulty filtration, and burning of indoor fuels.

Many of these are not new. The first air pollutants in history were most likely from fires warming the caves of early man. Burning wood, possibly the sweetest smell known to mankind, has its downside: it generates benzopyrenes and other hydrocarbons. Much later in time, newfound fossil fuels generated additional toxins: burning natural gas emits high amounts of carbon monoxide and nitrogen dioxide, whereas oil or coal generates sulfur dioxide.

According to the World Health Organization, traditional indoor stoves can increase respiratory infections, pulmonary disease, and lung cancer. In homes where biomass fuels and coal are used for cooking and heating, particulate matter levels may be 10–50 times higher than the guideline values. Frying or grilling foods as well creates particulate matter and other harmful compounds, a process of combustion that receives little attention.

Yet all of the poisonous by-products of fossil fuels have been around for a lot longer than Weight Watchers. Logic tells us then that these pollutants, while carcinogenic, are probably not to blame for the current obesity epidemic. What then?

Synthetic or man-made chemicals are new on the scene. Some add pounds. Those that promote obesity are called obesogens. Yet of the approximately 70,000 documented synthetic chemicals, only a few have been tested to determine their effects on weight.

Endocrine Disruptors

One class stands out in the lineup: those that interfere with complex endocrine systems.

These chemicals are called endocrine disrupting chemicals (EDCs) or endocrine disruptors. They have been defined by the Environmental Protection Agency (EPA) as "an exogenous agent that interferes with the production, release, transport, metabolism, binding, action, or elimination of natural hormones in the body responsible for the maintenance of homeostasis and the regulation of developmental processes."[6]

Quick review: an endocrine system involves glands that secrete hormones. These hormones travel from head to toe, dropping chemical messages on receptors. Insulin, for instance, squirts out of the pancreas and then calls the shots in sugar control throughout the body. And estrogen, primarily a female hormone, tinkers in countless places too. Chemicals that disturb an endocrine system are called "endocrine disruptors." (Note that "estrogen disruptors" are now folded into this broader class that includes androgens, progestins, and thyroid, hypothalamic, and pituitary hormones.)

Endocrine-disrupting compounds are hard to avoid. They are found in thousands of products: plastic storage containers, insect spray, lawn care items, cosmetics, and many industrial uses.

Bisphenol A (BPA) is the most notorious endocrine disruptor. It is everywhere in modern societies. BPA makes plastic harder and is used in cash register receipts. In addition to baby bottles and sippy cups, it is found in reusable food and drink containers, paints, adhesives, compact discs, DVDs, eyeglass lenses, sports safety goggles, and helmets. BPA can leak from plastic containers to contaminate foods, beverages, and drinking water. Despite initial synthesis in the late 1800s, BPA only emerged as a valuable compound in the plastics industry in the 1950s; today over 6 billion pounds are produced each year. Consequently, in over 95 percent of nearly 400 US adults and children urine samples tested by the CDC, BPA was found.[7]

How Endocrine Disruptors Harm

BPA is clever. It has more than one way to derail a healthy body. It binds to receptors in a chemical version of musical chairs where the normal hormone is shut out. And it can go both ways, juggling estrogen and androgens. BPA also disrupts the pancreas, which triggers insulin resistance. According to Newbold, BPA has potential for other biological bedlam at low exposure levels, including interfering with enzyme and neuron activity.

Remember, fat cells are dynamic living cells, constantly swapping signals with fellow fat cells as well as the brain, liver, stomach, pancreas, and more. It comes as no surprise then that fat cells fight back when caught in a sea of polluting chemicals.

In a journal article titled "Obesogens," Felix Grün explains what happens:

The environmental obesogen hypothesis postulates chemical pollutants that are able to promote obesity by altering homeostatic metabolic set-points, disrupting appetite controls, perturbing lipid homeostasis to promote adipocyte hypertrophy, or stimulating adipogenic pathways that enhance adipocyte hyperplasia during development or in adults.[8]

Simply put:

- our body struggles to keep weight higher (altered set point)
- more or longer hunger signals (disrupted appetite controls)
- larger fat cells (hypertrophy)
- more fat cells are made (hyperplasia)

How all this takes place is still being unraveled in labs across the world. Obesogens may target any of the critical steps, signals, and pathways that mobilize to maintain weight. They mess with the thyroid, the glucocorticoids, the hypothalamus, the pancreas, and more. With thousands of chemicals, the damage is done in different ways. Some are more weight-inducing at low than high exposures. This is a sore point between scientists in the field and chemical companies. Laura Vandenberg and colleagues wrote in 2012 *Endocrine Reviews* that "the effects of low doses cannot be predicted by the effects observed at high doses. Thus, fundamental changes in chemical testing and safety determination are needed to protect human health."[9] While tiny amounts of estrogen, testosterone, thyroid hormones, and other natural hormones have always been known to affect fetuses, it is not hard to make that leap to similar health effects from synthetic chemicals. Timing of exposure, gender, and genetic predisposition also figure in.[10]

A team led by Beverly Rubin at Tufts University Medical Center put BPA into the drinking water of rats from the sixth day of pregnancy through lactation. Those pups "exposed to BPA exhibited an increase in body weight that was apparent soon after birth and continued into adulthood."[11] New studies confirm the effect: weight rose in offspring of mothers exposed to BPA during gestation and lactation.[12]

In a study of children culled from government data sets, of those with high urinary levels of BPA, obesity was more likely—about twice as likely for the top quarter. The association was strong. The lead author of the study, pediatrician Leonardo Trasande of the New York University School of Medicine, told Nicholas Bakalar of the *New York Times* in 2012, "our study suggests the need to reconsider the decision not to ban BPA in food packaging."[13]

BPA is not the only endocrine disruptor—it is just one of the most studied because of the high volume in use. There could be thousands or more, some still unidentified. A review by Newbold suggests that many chemicals can cause weight gain: organochlorines; organophosphates; carbamates; polychlorinated biphenyls; polybrominated biphenyls; phthalates; perfluoroctanoic acid (PFOA); cadmium, lead, and arsenic; and solvents. With so many chemicals and so many ways for them to interfere—even at tiny doses—is it any wonder we are gaining weight?

Tobacco

Some people smoke to avoid eating too much. It's a little supermodel trick that backfires. After quitting, weight appears more quickly, as much due to metabolic changes as to increased munching to keep the mouth busy. Appetite also returns. So could smoking or quitting contribute to today's epidemic obesity?

Absolutely. One way is the above-mentioned metabolic swing caused by smoking. Nicotine reduces feeding in animals and weight in humans. After quitting, the metabolism shifts. Even gut microbes change, leaning toward the types more prevalent in obese people. Weight creeps up. In fact, the average weight gain in the long term after a smoker has quit is 7 kilograms or about 15 pounds.[14]

Whether secondhand smoke contributes to obesity is harder to gauge. Although living with a heavy smoker may expose you to asthma, heart disease, and cancer, little is known about its effects on obesity. Smokers and secondhand smokers in the same household do tend to be shorter, poorer, and less educated—other factors associated with increased rates of obesity—than nonsmokers, but blaming secondhand smoke may be misguided.

Household Products

Few women read ingredient labels on their mascaras or moisturizers. Probably because they can't: the words are indecipherable to the non-scientist, which is almost everyone. Yet recently the ingredients have come under fire from environmental groups. A review of the literature completed at the School of Medicine at Virginia Commonwealth University in the United States looked at common personal care product ingredients: phthalate esters, parabens, ultraviolet filters, polycyclic musks, and antimicrobials. The authors concluded: "Although select constituents exhibit interactions with the endocrine system in the laboratory, the evidence linking personal care products to endocrine disruptive effects in humans is for the most part lacking."[15] But these substances did show disruption "with the endocrine system in the laboratory," which is not exactly a vote of confidence.

While the United States Food and Drug Administration (FDA) does not regulate ingredients in cosmetics, it does require retailers to label the ingredients. Take a look at parabens, "the most widely used preservatives in cosmetics. . . . FDA believes that at the present time there is no reason for consumers to be concerned about the use of cosmetics containing parabens." Yet they include "important information for consumers who want to determine whether a product contains an ingredient they wish to avoid" on their website. This is some of that FDA information:

- "Cosmetics that may contain parabens include makeup, moisturizers, hair care products, and shaving products, among others."

- "Although parabens can act similarly to estrogen, they have been shown to have much less estrogenic activity than the body's naturally occurring estrogen."

- "The most common parabens used in cosmetic products are methylparaben, propylparaben, and butylparaben. Typically, more than one paraben is used in a product."[16]

Then there are phthalates which multitask: they are solvents, plasticizers, lubricants, and stabilizers. You will find them in a huge number of products such as toys, medical equipment, medications, cosmetics, and food packaging. So if you're a kid, a nurse, or a patient, or wear lipstick or eat, you've been exposed.

Several studies looked for an association between phthalates and obesity in humans. In analyzing NHANES data, the authors reported links between waist circumference and several phthalates in men.[17] And a more recent look at the same database showed a phthalate association with body mass index that also varied by age and gender.[18]

Other chemicals being studied are ultraviolet filters in sunscreens; polycyclic musks in fragrance and deodorants; and antimicrobials such as triclosan used in antibacterial soaps, toothpaste, and medical equipment. Our personal care products may be doing more harm than good.

INNERMOST AIR: THE WOMB

Pregnant women are extremely cautious. They don't drink, smoke, or color their hair. They don't bungee jump, skydive, or ride without seat belts.

But they do slather on suntan lotions, drink from sports bottles, use hand sanitizers, paint the nursery, shave with scented gels, reheat in plastic bowls, fertilize the garden, spray with air freshener, and live with smokers.

The babies they carry are under siege from chemicals. Though adults also suffer, the unborn are extremely fragile. First, the fetus doesn't have the protective mechanisms which an adult has: fully developed DNA repair tools, a capable immune system, detoxifying enzymes, complete liver metabolism, and a fully functional blood-brain barrier. Chemicals can pass through the placenta. And worse, the fetus has a fast metabolism, which can add to toxicity.[19] When cells divide rapidly while being exposed to chemicals, things go wrong. Their marching orders are altered. And these changes, including tendency to obesity, may not appear until adulthood. Or even scarier, the damages may show up way down the road, in the cells of future generations. Genes are altered.

Yes, that BPA in your water bottle may figure strongly in your great-grandchild's life. You may be exposing all your future generations to obesity based on your contact with chemicals. Quite a legacy.

Incredibly, companies in the United States often don't have to provide safety data for chemicals. It is up to the government to assess risk. Data do exist though. Animal studies usually clear the way for manufacturers when little harm comes to the animal even at high doses. Remember hearing that you'd have to have 100 diet colas a day to get the same dose of cyclamates that caused cancer in rats? Studies typically test high dose levels and a common outcome of such toxicity is weight *loss*. These findings may be deceiving, however, since very low doses can be harmful in their own ways, one of which may be obesity.[20] How do these pollutants do their damage? As mentioned with indoor air, these chemicals are called endocrine disruptors.

Take a look at how one widely used estrogen caused obesity. If you are a woman over 70 years of age, it may be familiar.

Diethylstilbestrol (DES), though no longer used to prevent miscarriage, was used in up to eight million pregnancies worldwide until 1971. Many of the offspring are now in their forties and fifties. Exposure in the womb is associated with obesity later in life. High prenatal DES doses caused lower birth weight followed by a "catch-up period" that led to obesity, but low doses with no impact on birth weight still resulted in obesity later on in life. The "catch-up" phase is critical. This is the phenomenon seen in countries exposed to famine: inadequate nutrition in the womb causes compensation later in life, which results in obesity.[21]

Another worry is that DES is also linked to diabetes development. DES-treated mice had altered glucose metabolism. While the ban on the use of DES is welcomed, in light of its role in the obesity epidemic, considerable harm has already been done.

BPA, however, is still produced in massive quantities: more than 800 million kilograms annually in the United States alone. No wonder BPA finds its way into the womb. Measurable BPA levels have been reported in human urine, serum, breast milk, maternal and fetal plasma, amniotic fluid, and placental tissues. Humans are widely exposed to BPA and it appears to amass in the fetus.

Rats and mice get fat when low BPA doses are added to their fetal and newborn space. How does this happen? BPA increases fat cells, causes insulin resistance, and bumps up release of inflammatory factors relevant to obesity and the metabolic syndrome.[22]

Here's another suspect chemical: perfluorooctanoic acid (PFOA) is the magical coating that keeps food from sticking to pans. Unfortunately, PFOA is also a chemical that may play a role in obesity later in life. In addition to nonstick pans, it is used in microwave popcorn bags, stain-resistant carpets, cleaning solutions, and some clothing. It can be found in everyone's blood, and that includes polar bears and pandas at the farthest reaches of the planet. Industrial runoff and trash disposal contaminate soil and drinking water. Fish from polluted waters have especially high amounts. In animal studies, PFOA can cause cancer, physical development delays, endocrine disruption, and early death.

Now a 2012 report has linked this common chemical with human obesity. Over twenty years ago, researchers in Denmark measured levels of PFOA in 665 pregnant women. Recently they looked at their offspring as young adults. The women, but not men, were three times as likely to be heavier with larger waists than those who had lower levels.[23]

The good news is that the companies using PFOA have pledged to eliminate them from products by 2015. But damage has been done.[24]

Transgenerational harm is also evident in tributyltins (TBT), compounds in the organotin group. Humans are exposed through contaminated seafood and shellfish, fungicides on crops, and antifungal agents in wood treatments, industrial water systems, and textiles. TBT exposure in mice before birth caused them to gain more fat later in life.[25] In 2013, scientists at the University of California, Irvine found that those pregnant mice that were fed TBT birthed pups with bigger fat cells and more of them. Most disturbingly, the children and grandchildren of these mice inherited the fat changes in spite of never having been exposed to the chemical. TBT alters genes, which sets future generations up for lifelong struggles with weight.[26]

The Youngest Secondhand Smokers

Smoking cigarettes anytime while pregnant will make a fatter child by age ten. This finding came from a study that followed over 10,000 pregnant women and their offspring in Bristol, England.[27]

Backing this up was a look at data based on 84,563 children whose mothers smoked during pregnancy; they also were more likely to be overweight.[28]

And another: With 369 Spanish children born in 1997–1998, smoking in the first trimester was more strongly associated with overweight than smoking later in pregnancy.[29]

These were some possible explanations:

- Mothers who smoke may feed their underweight newborn more.

- Smokers eat differently than nonsmokers so their children may also.

- Physical activity may be lower in children of smokers.

- Nicotine passes through the placenta, reduces appetite and body weight while in the womb, but then compensates with more hunger and weight gain later.[30]

While many women quit smoking before or when they learn they are pregnant, many continue. Over 10 percent in the United States continue to smoke, putting their offspring at risk for future obesity and other complications.[31]

Women who smoked while pregnant were more likely to be younger, shorter, less educated, and from lower socioeconomic classes. They did not breastfeed, introduced their child to solids earlier, and had shorter partners and lighter babies.[32] The culture surrounding smoking may also be a fast track to obesity.

OUTDOOR AIR

I had been warned about the *khamsein* in Egypt: a blizzard of sand and dust and cement with a few geckos mixed in. A khamsein whirls and burns your eyes and your ears, and can even seep inside a bedroom closet in some type of messy wizardry. This can't be healthy. Cairo is polluted in many ways—burning trash, burning rubber, and burning rice fields, along with noxious car exhaust and smoldering cigarettes—but other cities are worse. The World Bank reported in 2010 that 16 of the world's top 20 most polluted cities are in China. Linfen City in Shanxi Province, China, which is known for its coal industry, was the world's most polluted.

Developed countries are polluted too.

Despite decades of cleanup measures, the American Lung Association State of the Air 2012 revealed that nearly half the population of the United States "still suffer pollution levels that are often dangerous to breathe." The report found that unhealthy air posed a threat to the lives and health of "over 127 million people—[roughly] 41 percent of the nation."[33] Even cities like Salt Lake City, Utah, and North Pole, Alaska, which sound pristine, are choking with pollution—the first from automobiles and industry and the latter from burning coal and wood for warmth. At times the air quality readings in North Pole are twice as bad as that of Beijing, according to Kim Murphy writing in the *Los Angeles Times* in 2013.[34]

Air is judged by ozone and particulate matter. Greenhouse gases including carbon dioxide, methane, and nitrous oxide are bad for respiratory systems, according to the EPA. But a new slyer villain has emerged: the small bits, called particulate matter (PM).

According to the World Health Organization, PM affects more people than any other pollutant. PM is a jumble of solids, liquids, and organic and inorganic matter: mostly sulfate, nitrates, ammonia, sodium chloride, carbon, mineral dust, and water. The smaller particulates at 2.5 µm are most dangerous because they easily invade the lungs.[35]

And as you may have guessed by the recipe, these PM2.5s, which emerge from burning fuels, are linked to asthma, lung cancer, and other respiratory diseases. People exposed to pollution don't live as long. The mortality in cities with high levels of pollution exceeds that observed in relatively cleaner cities by 15 to 20 percent.

The link to obesity is new. How could this happen? The idea is that PM contributes to insulin resistance and adipose inflammation. In one experiment, mice exposed to PM2.5 showed insulin resistance and more visceral fat and inflammation among other defects.[36]

And in a joint Harvard-MIT study, researchers concluded that PM2.5 may contribute to increased diabetes in the adult US population, adding to the mounting evidence in that regard.[37]

Outdoor air presents other dangers. Just as indoors, hazardous endocrine disruptors are also used outdoors. Chemicals known as human endocrine disruptors include heavy metals, solvents, organophosphates, phthalates, dioxins, pesticides, and butyltins.

Let's begin with one chemical that has been banned but may have contributed to the obesity problem: Dichlorodiphenyltrichloroethane, or DDT, a widely used pesticide which won its maker a Nobel Prize, has been linked to many cancers and is a known endocrine disruptor and neurotoxin. Besides its successful use in fighting malaria and typhus, DDT was the active ingredient in many aerosol bug sprays and home lawn sprays. It went into plastic shelf linings and home carpets. By the late 1950s, the world was awash in DDT.[38] Unfortunately, DDT has been shown to act as an endocrine disruptor in numerous studies.

Despite a near global ban today, we still have to worry. DDT left something behind for future generations: Dichlorodiphenyldichloroethylene, or DDE, a by-product, persists in the environment, especially soil. Exposure to DDT and DDE occurs mostly from eating foods particularly meat, fish, and poultry. DDE can be detected in fat, blood, urine, semen, and breast milk.[39]

In a 2011 study, prenatal DDE exposure was associated with rapid weight gain in the first six months and elevated body mass index later in infancy, among infants of normal-weight mothers.[40]

Organochlorine chemicals, of which DDT and DDE are members, are widely used in agriculture and industry. One of these, hexachlorobenzene, was measured in umbilical cord blood at birth. The levels correlated with overweight in children at six years of age. These children were exposed in the womb.[41]

Organophosphates also cause obesity in animals.[42] And organotins are another class that affect fat cells and body weight.[43]

But wait, here is more disturbing news: our fat doubles as a toxic waste dump. White adipose tissue (WAT) stockpiles persistent organic pollutants (POPs), which are hard to degrade.[44] These tough-guy POPs are endocrine disruptors, associated with the metabolic syndrome and type 2 diabetes. And in one recent study from Belgium, blood levels of POPs were linked to obesity.[45] They can also be shuffled to the developing fetus. The list of POPs includes tributyltin, DDT, and many of the organochlorine class.

WATER

As countries struggle to improve air, water is getter worse.

Poor water quality and bad sanitation are deadly; the WHO estimates that safe water could prevent 1.4 million child deaths from diarrhea each year.[46] In the developing world, much wastewater still goes untreated into local rivers and streams. But even when treated, pollution can be created across the chain: when disposing and burning of treated sewage sludge, using sludge as fertilizer, and treating toxic waste.

And just as we can't escape breathing air, we need water. Disguised as lemonade or coffee, we're still drinking water. Boil it, filter it, sweeten it—you still have water that has toxins or remnants of something you may not choose to be drinking. Or bathing in or swimming in, for that matter. Alarm bells should sound when our lakes and rivers offer up bizarre stories like these: fish with no interest in sex, frogs sprouting extra legs, and male alligators—in polluted Lake Apopka in Florida—growing penises half the normal size.

In the Potomac watershed near Washington, DC, male smallmouth bass have rapidly transformed into "intersex fish" that display female characteristics. Researchers found female germ cells (oocytes) in the testes of more than 80 percent of the male smallmouth bass. "There must be something in the water"—long a whimsical aside—has become a disturbing reality.

The "somethings" in the water are endocrine disruptors—and a whole slew of other toxins, many capable of adding to the obesity problem. The suspects confusing the smallmouth bass inside the beltway? Birth control pills and antibacterial soap in sewage as well as runoff from farms, which brings pesticides and animal hormones, according to David Fahrenthold writing in the *Washington Post.*[47]

Different agencies in different countries safeguard the health of their people through laws and regulatory agencies. Agencies set standards of allowable maximums.

In the United States, the EPA regulates tap water while the Food and Drug Administration regulates bottled water. Surveys show that people drink bottled water because they think it is safer. Is bottled water safer than water from a tap? Sorry, there is no easy answer because it depends on which bottle and which tap.

"Neither the public nor federal regulators know nearly enough about where bottled water comes from and what safeguards are in place to ensure its safety," said Representative Bart Stupak, chairman of the oversight committee of the US House Energy and Commerce Committee in 2009.[48]

Here's a brief look at types of pollutants in our water supply condensed from EPA publications.

- Microorganisms: These are primarily from fecal waste. Examples are Giardia, which can cause gastrointestinal diseases with vomiting and diarrhea, and Legionnaires, which causes pneumonia and coliforms, including the ubiquitous *E. coli*.

- Disinfectants: Chlorine and chlorine oxides used to control microbes can cause eye irritation, anemia, and nervous disorders.

- Disinfectant By-products: Bromates, chlorites, and other disinfectants for the water are linked to cancer and anemia in certain levels. Bladder cancer has been associated with exposure to chlorination by-products in drinking water.

- Inorganic chemicals: From antimony and arsenic to thallium (not quite A to Z but numerous nonetheless), this group is frightening in its possibilities. We have mercury, lead, chromium, cyanide—the usual bad actors—plus many more. For example, chronic exposure to arsenic has the potential to cause wide ranges of carcinogenic and non-carcinogenic health effects such as cancer of the skin and internal organs, diabetes mellitus, hypertension, and respiratory conditions.

- Organic chemicals: With longer, more exotic names, these are just as dangerous as the metallica in the inorganic club. Organic and inorganic differ only in the fact that the first group contains carbon, a tidbit of high school chemistry that has come in handy.

- Radionuclides: Natural erosion processes create alpha particle contamination, which can lead to cancers.

Some of the above, such as mercury and lead, are celebrity pollutants (the latter thought to have felled the Roman empire[49]) eating up the research dollars, whereas the shy ones may be just as harmful and factor into the obesity epidemic. Deciding safe levels for many thousands of chemicals is the daunting if not impossible task facing regulators.

The EPA is screening over 200 chemicals to determine endocrine effects, namely their ability to mimic estrogen, androgen, and thyroid hormone actions. Unfortunately, as the regulators decide which ones are harmful, they continue to be widely used in agricultural and industry. Many of the tens of thousands of chemicals in use have never been tested for safety.

One obvious source of endocrine disruptors in our water supply is the real thing. Not Coke, though we will have to look into that, but actual estrogens from oral contraceptives. The birth control pill was introduced to the American market in 1960 after Margaret Sanger convinced Planned Parenthood to fund development. Almost 12 million women in the United States alone take the pill, and their urine contains the hormone. Some research says that birth control pills account for less than 1 percent of the estrogens found in the nation's drinking water supplies. Knowing that sewage treatment plants remove virtually all of the main estrogen—17 alpha-ethinylestradiol (EE2)—in oral contraceptives, the scientists decided to pin down the main sources of estrogens in water supplies.

Their report suggests that most hormones enter drinking water supplies from other sources. According to research cited here, "animal manure accounts for 90 percent of estrogens in the environment."[50]

Other drugs in water cause weight gain. In 2006, researchers at the Mario Negri Institute for Pharmacological Research in Milan looked at pollution by pharmaceuticals in Italy. Humans as well as animals using veterinary drugs are the major sources. The authors found that while "sewage system[s] [are] important . . . in the control of contamination, [they] are not able efficiently to abate a substantial part of water-borne pharmaceuticals."[51]

Some argue that such minuscule amounts are harmless. Except now scientists are finding that small doses can also disrupt metabolisms. How do we fix this?

SOLUTIONS

Short of living in a tent—make it untreated canvas with no synthetic threads—on a mountaintop far from civilization, what can be done to limit our exposure to obesogenic pollution?

Let's start with indoor air, a place we may think is under our control yet can be surprisingly toxic.

Indoors

Nothing is lovelier than a crackling fire in the hearth, right? Well, as comforting as it seems, wood emits carbon monoxide, smoke, and particulate matter. Pressed logs may be a cleaner alternative.

Some computer printers spew harmful particles. One solution is to set up the printer in a ventilated part of the house and stand away while printing. Color ink is more harmful than black and white.

Dirt in the form of pesticides, animal waste, and other trash is carried in on the soles of our shoes. Do as many Europeans and Asians do—leave those shoes by the door.

Dry cleaning clothing is a problem. Harmful volatile organic compounds (VOCs) from the cleaning chemicals invade your indoor environment. If you must go this route, air out well before hanging up in your closet. Many carpets and paints are also laced with VOCs.

Cash register receipts are rife with BPA. They can be refused. Take only the ones you will keep for your records.

Plastic is a big challenge. Think about this: "The quantity of plastics produced in the first 10 years of the current century is likely to approach the quantity produced in the entire century that preceded."[52] Plastics of course are invaluable in many ways, in medical technology, computers, and packaging.

What's wrong with plastic? Plastic is made from oil—an unsustainable source—and it takes many lifetimes for one plastic bag to dissolve. It breaks down into smaller and smaller petrochemicals. When it rains, each plastic bag tossed in sewers or dumps becomes an ideal breeding ground for mosquitos, one factor in the malaria epidemic. Bangladesh was one of the first to ban plastic bags because major floods ensued after drains were blocked. Many other countries and cities followed with either a tax or outright ban.

Bisphenol A (BPA)—a proven obesogen—is found in many commercial products including lightweight plastics. The European Union banned the use of BPA from plastic baby bottles starting in 2011, while the United States banned it in baby bottles a year later. Some manufacturers are phasing out BPA; Tupperware's website says it does not use BPA in children's products sold in the United States and Canada.

Government toxicology scientists say that to reduce exposure, people can avoid non-recyclable plastic containers that have the #7 in the recycle triangle because they may contain BPA. Plastic labeled #3 may contain phthalates as well as BPA. Plastics with recycling codes 1, 2, 4 and 5 are thought to be safer. Avoid using these plastics in the microwave, and don't wash them in the dishwasher with harsh detergents.

- Discard scratched baby bottles and infant feeding cups as they may release BPA.

- To mix powdered infant formula, heat liquids in a BPA-free container.

- Breastfeed, if possible.

- With cosmetics, lotions, and toiletries, reading labels is a must. Avoid products with parabens and all its cousins: methylparaben, propylparaben and butylparaben. Better yet, opt for simplicity in personal care. Baking soda works well as a teeth cleaner, and olive oil is safe as a hair conditioner and moisturizer.

- Avoid phthalates when buying toys, cosmetics, and packaging.

- Limit perfumes and deodorants that have polycyclic musks.

- Rather than use suntan lotions, cover up with hats and long sleeves and try to avoid the sun at peak hours.

- When painting, either a room or a portrait, ventilate well.

- Avoid air fresheners. Put some cinnamon sticks in a pot of water or buy fresh flowers.

- Decorate with green plants, which gobble up your carbon dioxide.

- Rethink hand sanitizers. Triclosan may be more dangerous than a stray microbe.

- Wash fruits and vegetables well to get rid of residuals herbicides and pesticides.

- Cook with cast iron instead of nonstick pans, and microwave in glass.

- Eat few processed foods.

- Use a kitchen fan to vent cooking fumes and vapors to the outside. And use the fan over the stove while cooking.

- And finally, if anyone smokes in your home, ask him or her to take it outside.

Outdoors

- Exercise indoors when pollution indexes are dangerous.

- Take public transportation or walk.

- Wear a mask if biking in a city.

- Advocate for clear air. Don't litter.

- Use green pesticides on your garden. Use alternative

weed management such as planting cover crops, rotating crops and using mechanical weed control methods.

Water

- Call your local government for a report on your water source.

- If using well water, test it annually.

- Wash your clothes less often; they will last longer.

Consider installing a water filter to remove metals and some bacteria. According to an article in *Scientific America* online, "Of the many different kinds of in-home water filtration systems available today, only those employing reverse osmosis have been shown to effectively filter out some drugs. Some makers of activated carbon water filters claim their products catch pharmaceuticals, but independent research has not verified such claims."[53] Do not use toilets or sinks to dispose of unused medications.

These chemicals are not the cause of all obesity, of course. But for younger generations who have been awash in chemicals from every source, even before birth, they may be one reason.

Clearly, fighting obesity is not as simple as portion control and getting off the couch.

4

· · · ·

SUBURBAN LEGENDS: SPRAWL & OBESITY

Suburbia with its wide-open spaces was supposed to make us healthy. Now it seems the opposite is true.

VANI LIVES IN A PALATIAL HOME IN THE KATAMEYA development on the outskirts of Cairo. The marbled three-story foyer and swooping stairways wouldn't be out of place in an upscale shopping mall or a Sotheby advertisement. The view from the patio, beyond the pool, reveals carpets of plush lawn rimmed with blooming bougainvillea, which lead on to a designer golf course dotted with palm trees and fountains. Who wouldn't want to live in such splendor? But luxury, she admits, has a price beyond a massive monthly bill: In order to reach her son's school or shop for food or meet friends for lunch, Vani crosses nearly 20 kilometers (about 12 miles) of desert and asphalt, a trip which traps her in a car for two to three hours every day. What once looked like the Promised Land now looks like no man's land.

Equally ambitious but a touch less Disney, a project named 6th of October City relocated thousands of Egyptian to the desert, their chance to live in better housing conditions. Soon, however, the new residents realized that trekking back to Cairo for work was not only difficult but also expensive given the bus and taxi fees added to already limited budgets. And not surprisingly, the sociable Cairenes missed the pulse of the city. Many have moved back. Yet the building continues. In this city of 20 million, suburbs and the even more far-flung exurbs are rising out of the desert at a frightening pace. The only way out is by car on traffic-choked roadways.

Across the globe, similar lapses in vision have fostered the same wrong-headed development: lush oases of housing are isolated and left unconnected to work, services, and even schools. Unlike many neighborhoods built before 1950 in the grid design, these new "neighborhoods built after 1970 tend[ed] to have a 'loops and lollipops' design."[1] Sidewalks are rare. Long trips in automobiles are mandatory. Decades later, the promise of suburbia has given way to reality. Once blinded by pretty lawns and walk-in closets and other amenities of McMansions, homeowners are waking up to the ugly truth of long commutes and its side effects. It all seemed so perfect. Until it wasn't.

As we shall see, of the many good things that were supposed to happen in the suburbs, there were unintended consequences. Obesity was one of them. From Cairo to Los Angeles to Mumbai to Shanghai to Sydney, sprawl is an unhealthy reality.

BIRTH OF SPRAWL

Sprawl: "to spread or develop irregularly or without restraint."[2]

That's the Merriam-Webster definition. The version used in academic circles, courtesy of sprawl expert Russ Lopez: "an overall pattern of development across a metropolitan area where large percentages of the population live in lower-density residential areas."[3] Still the definition itself displays a measure of randomness. Other descriptions should be considered, such as a leapfrog-type development that when viewed from an airplane looks like an unfinished quilt and from the ground—a modern suburb.

America's first suburb was created in 1814 when a ferry steamed across the East River to Brooklyn from Manhattan. Trains and trolleys also stretched the distances people could travel between home and work. But what really put the sprawl in suburbia was the automobile. Beginning in the 1920s and exploding in the prosperous postwar years, automobile ownership allowed more Americans to live in the suburbs.[4] General Motors went to work dismantling streetcars, a popular form of public transport in most cities until the 1940s, and replacing tracks with smooth road and an assembly line of new cars. Another push came from the Federal Highway Act of 1956, signed by Dwight D. Eisenhower to construct 41,000 miles (66,000 km) of highways at a cost of 25 billion dollars. It was the biggest public works project in history, which made crossing long distances by automobile a reality.[5]

At the end of that road, the American dream sold by Madison Avenue lived in big houses separated from neighbors by moats of green lawns and tall fences. Downtowns were abandoned to those unfortunates who couldn't afford the house or the car needed to get to it. And in another blow to urban living, retailers left en masse to chase the money in the suburbs, setting up shop in strip malls or megamalls connected only by concrete highways. Public transportation lost its appeal and in many places was left to the huddled masses, the lower socioeconomic classes. Some inner cities became wastelands. Moreover, policy makers rewarded the automobile industry with tax incentives, and much later, from 2008 to 2010, bailouts and cash-for-clunker programs that would boost the country economically. But the lack of vision in built environments has not only greatly increased our dependence on fossil fuels and foreign oil, with its threats to the environment and national security, but it has made automobile ownership mandatory in the suburbs. And why is that a problem? Who, after all, doesn't enjoy a ride on the open road, music blasting and hair blowing in the breeze? In truth, the downsides are many: greenhouse gas emissions; high costs of ownership; traffic deaths and injuries—which occur disproportionately to the young—isolation for the old and the young who don't drive; and a downside that is the focus of this book: obesity.

To be sure, the automobile is just one villain of many in this saga of sprawl. Real estate developers bought up huge tracts of farmland and open space cheaply and then created housing that gave a lot more house for the money, provided it was situated far enough away from any urban area. Zoning laws from local governments limited mixed-use housing, ostensibly to protect communities from pollution and noise of industry. The outcome was that vital services including supermarkets and hospitals were separated from homes, a trend that has proven unhealthy. Politicians vowed to get everyone in a house they owned, and renting became stigmatized as personal economic failure. Lending regulations were eased and banks and mortgage companies spat out loans as if they had no stake in their repayment, which turned out to be true; they simply bundled them and sold them off after taking a nice slice of profit. When the easy money started bidding wars for houses, a seller's market created a bubble that pushed people farther and farther out to the suburbs to find something affordable. The average home in Manhattan cost well over one million dollars in 2013.

While the average worker in New York City spent 44 minutes commuting, the rest of Americans posted average commute times of 25 minutes.[6] Even though it is 63 miles from Los Angeles, Palmdale is considered a bedroom community. From a population of about 12,000 in 1980, Palmdale with its affordable housing has grown to over 150,000 today, with many residents making the long commute daily to work in Los Angeles.[7]

Researcher Russ Lopez at the Boston University School of Public Health used the 2000 US Census data to create an index that measured urban sprawl on the basis of density and compactness.[8] In an important paper, Lopez pinpointed the causes of urban sprawl: "affluence that enables households to purchase larger houses on larger lots, cultural values that reject urban living and emphasize automobile use, inexpensive land values that support urban sprawl–dependent lifestyles, and government policies that promote urban sprawl."[9]

Much of the world has succumbed to sprawl. A spin around Google Earth reveals that virtually all countries are seeing suburbs and exurbs arise far from schools, workplaces, and vital services. Satellite imagery showed that all of the 120 cities sampled around the globe are beginning to spread.

Sprawl is on the rise. Obesity is on the rise. Could they be connected?

HOW SPRAWL MAKES US FAT

It's no surprise that researchers at the University of Maryland are studying the relationship between sprawl and obesity. The campus, home to more than 35,000, draws its students from across the state spread between Baltimore and Washington, DC, and beyond. This 2006 study looked at the connection between urban sprawl and body mass index (BMI), which is weight in kilograms divided by metric height squared. Data from the 1997 National Longitudinal Survey of Youth were used.[10]

The results? In both groups, adolescents (aged 12–17) and young adults (aged 18–23), being overweight or at risk of overweight was associated with county sprawl. Young adults living in more compact counties were presumably "more active in their routine daily activities. While not classified as formal 'exercise,' they may walk to lunch rather than drive, walk up stairs in a multistory environment, or take transport to work that requires a walk at one or both ends," surmised the authors. The relationship between sprawl and overweight for youth actually proved stronger than that between sprawl and obesity for adults in the original study by Reid Ewing and colleagues.[11] This is considered a "cross-sectional" study. In another type of study termed "longitudinal," the same individuals are studied over a span of time. In this case, the question was asked: did BMI change when individuals moved between counties, with varying rates of sprawl? No, sprawl was not related.

Some solid studies link urban sprawl and obesity. Lopez found associations between urban sprawl and overweight and obesity.[12] And when conducting research at Rutgers University, Ewing and his team found that residents of sprawling counties weighed more, walked less during leisure time, and had higher blood pressures than those in compact counties. More than 200,000 adults from across the United States were pooled for the survey.[13] In 2002, the Centers for Disease Control and Prevention (CDC) released a report that also connected urban sprawl and obesity.[14]

And when researchers looked at over 1200 residents from 120 neighborhoods in Portland, Oregon, each 10-percent rise in land-use mix was linked to a 25-percent drop in overweight and obesity. Blending residential, commercial, and industrial areas translated into more physical activity. Putting homes next to stores and offices makes perfect sense.[15]

Here's another angle, this one across a wide swath of time and place: scientists at the Institute for Health Research and Policy in Chicago considered the impact of urban sprawl between 1970 and 2000 on obesity of residents in metropolitan areas across the United States. Results? As population density fell, obesity rose. The researchers concluded that "estimates indicate that if the average metropolitan area had not experienced the decline in the proportion of population living in dense areas over the last 30 years, the rate of obesity would have been reduced by approximately 13%."[16]

Hindsight is not always easy.

Australians also worry about sprawl. Sydney, Australia's largest city with a population over four million, is seeing substantial growth, in both suburbs and obesity. Using population density, scientists there have found that sprawling suburbs meant more obesity as well as too little activity.[17] Rates of obesity in Australia rival those in the United States.

And consider Mississippi, which has the unfortunate distinction of being the fattest state in the United States. It is also home to an alarming amount of sprawl. Lopez wrote: "Many of the metropolitan areas that have the highest levels of urban sprawl are located in the South. This association was one of the first links between levels of urban sprawl and the risk for being obese or overweight."[18] It is just such an environment, added Lopez, that breeds obesity: sources of high-calorie food, poor street patterns, lack of pedestrian amenities, difficult-to-access destinations, and neighborhood perceptions.

At its simplest, obesity is an imbalance of energy in and energy out. Many factors tip the scales toward excessive calorie storage. Sprawl is one of them and worse, sprawl can upset both sides of the equation.

Energy In: The type and amount of food eaten is affected by the neighborhood. For example, a shorter distance to supermarkets translates into more fruits and vegetables on plates in early research.[19] On the other hand, being close to fast-food restaurants spurs high-fat diets and higher BMIs.[20] Drive-thrus often outnumber supermarkets in the suburbs. And then there is the matter of cost; prices of healthy foods like tomatoes and broccoli go up as farmland is carved into suburbs. Potato chips and soda become bargains.

Energy Out: Physical activity spends energy. But why do people in suburbs move less?[21] Cul-de-sacs, wide lawns and like-minded neighbors promised a carefree playground of sports and fun activities. Backyard touch football and pickup basketball were going to replace the cultural amenities they had left behind in the city. It hasn't worked out that way. People drive their kids to sports practices and games. Soccer moms are legendary in the United States for the number of hours they spend inside their vehicles. According to a website run by Sierra Club, the oldest environmental group in the United States, sprawl lengthens trips and forces us to drive everywhere, even for a newspaper or a carton of milk. And as we saw in the previous chapter, pollution from cars is damaging to our health and can contribute to obesity. The average American driver currently spends the equivalent of 55 eight-hour workdays behind the wheel every year. Food shopping in the suburbs, a daily event in a city, is a marathon session miles away at big box stores. Costco and Walmart now capture a hefty share of the food dollar in the United States. Places of employment are even farther away from homes in the suburbs with some daily commutes adding ten hours or more of sitting time to the work week. School buses pick up kids and drop them off near their houses. And as for the extras such as a movie on Friday, mall on Saturday, and church on Sunday: nothing is within walking distance.

What is "walking distance?" This could be one mile for you or a mere block for your neighbor. The distance will vary depending on age, nationality, income, health, weather, time available, and a host of other variables. But one thing is clear: sprawl severely stretches walking distances.

People walk less when faced with space, as was seen in the Rutgers study.[22] One analyst tried to put a number on it: walking kicks in at densities between 1,000 and 3,999 persons per square mile.

Which traits encourage walking and physical activity? Individuals walk more when neighborhoods have more people, sidewalks, and streets that connect to many streets, shops, restaurants, doctors, and other destinations. Buses and trains offer some walking since passengers will have to get to the stop. Research indicates, "Urban sprawl may reduce the amount of time available for physical activity because parks or fitness facilities are more distant." Of course, not all suburban dwellers exercise less. Many bike and run and head to local parks to play sports, but often by car.[23]

Lopez explains it well: "Perhaps urban sprawl affects the propensity to walk, bike, or be otherwise physically active. People in high-sprawled areas may drive more. It has been hypothesized that urban form may influence the mixture of transportation modes used by a population. The pattern of streets in a neighborhood may affect how people use their cars and their propensity to walk."[24]

More sprawl means more driving. A report by Smart Growth documented the link between urban sprawl and more driving.[25] And according to the Harvard Alumni Health Study, "more than 50 studies . . . have examined the built environment and utilitarian travel."[26] Walking and bicycling for transportation were consistently associated with less sprawling communities.[27] A recent study reported that persons living in "walkable neighborhoods" walked more (34%) and drove less (26 miles/day) than those preferring and living in car-dependent neighborhoods (3% walked; 43 miles/day driven).[28]

Driving leads to obesity in several ways. The first obviously is because of less exercise. But cars also mean air pollution and added stress, both of which can add pounds.

Berlin is a city that has its share of sprawl, an exodus prompted after the wall fell in 1989. But the core of the city is a remarkable model of urban planning. A sophisticated web of subways, bus lanes and light-rail tracks supply convenient transport for every citizen. And as Germans are renowned for their love of the outdoors, they allowed forests to blanket one-third of the city, making raw nature accessible to everyone, even those without vehicles. Bicycle lanes crisscross the city. No car is needed to live in Berlin.

China was once a land of bikes and walkers. No more. Because of rapid economic advances, many millions of Chinese people are buying cars and motorcycles for the first time. Researchers at the University of North Carolina at Chapel Hill decided that the drastic shifts in transport patterns in China provided an ideal opportunity to see if there was a link between vehicle ownership and obesity. Fourteen percent of households in their study bought a motorized vehicle between 1989 and 1997. "Compared with those whose vehicle ownership did not change, men who [had] a vehicle [had gained] 1.8 kilograms [or nearly four pounds] more than the others." In addition, "the odds of being obese were 80 percent higher for men and women in households who owned a car or a motorcycle compared with those who did not own a vehicle."[29]

Sprawl causes obesity. Period. Well, if it were that simple we could all abandon the cul-de-sacs and move back to the cities. But just because urban sprawl is associated with obesity doesn't mean it causes obesity, say some critics. There are a number of gray areas.

For example, do active people choose places more conducive to walking?

Does the environment change the activity level of the individual or does the individual choose a neighborhood with lots of opportunities for physical exercise?

While there is a link between less sprawl and more walking, data show this: men who moved from more to less sprawling counties didn't walk more. Nor did their BMIs drop. This supports a theory advanced by Lopez that the causal association between urban sprawl and obesity is in the reverse direction: People who are already #10 overweight may choose to move to areas with greater levels of urban sprawl because they may find it easier to avoid walking. Climbing into a Dodge truck is less taxing than climbing up a fourth-floor walk-up in New York City. Self-selection bias may affect the type of people living in sprawling areas.

Still other studies, such as the 1997 US National Longitudinal Study of Youth (NLSY), saw links between more sprawl and higher BMI.[30] And unlike other results, one showed significant association between moving to less-sprawling counties and decreased BMI. There was also some self-selection: persons with lower BMI were more likely to move to less sprawling counties.[31] A problem here is that many studies have relied on subject's perception of their physical environment.[32] Active persons may be more aware of places to exercise, or they may be more willing to walk farther to their destinations.

Some of the discrepancies among the results may be due to the differences in the way that urban sprawl is measured.

In the Australian study,[33] for example, the authors found mixed results when looking at data for connections between sprawl and obesity:

> We used population density as our measure of urban sprawl. Lopez[34] created a sprawl index for metropolitan areas in the USA using population density at the census tract level whereas others have used the sprawl index created by Ewing et al.,[35] a metropolitan and county sprawl index derived from principal components analysis based on residential density, land-use mix, degree of centering, and street accessibility from a number of data sources such as the US Census, American Housing Survey, and the US Census Transportation Planning. We were unable to apply this alternative method of calculating the sprawl index to metropolitan Sydney because most of the required variables such as the percentage of residents with businesses or institutions within half a block from their home and the percentage of blocks 1/100 of a square mile or less in size are not routinely collected in Australia.

A third gray area is this: many inner city residents are obese.

While the suburbs may breed inactivity and excess calories, it is undeniable that many residents living in the inner city—an environment without the negative attributes of sprawl—are obese. This is true despite high densities, connecting streets and loads of sidewalks—all those positives that encourage fitness. This would seem to contradict the "sprawl as a cause of obesity" theory.

But remember, obesity has many partners.

Income, race, gender, and age all impact obesity.

For example, more affluent people may be able to afford healthier food. Poor people may live in food deserts, where junk food is cheap and wholesome food expensive. (More on this in the chapter on access.) Poverty is certainly a contributor. Using data from the 1990–1994 National Health Interview Survey, researchers found that adults residing in neighborhoods with a high concentration of poverty and in neighborhoods with a high percentage of blacks were more likely to be obese.[36]

In trying to explain the higher body mass index of black adults in the United States, other researchers looked at both socioeconomic status and community disadvantage. They found both were related to higher BMI among women but not among men.[37]

In a 2008 study, researchers looked at the influence of neighborhood on the weight status of adults 55 years and older. An alarming 70 percent of this group is overweight in the United States. "Eight neighbohood scales [were considered]: economic advantage, economic disadvantage, air pollution, crime and segregation, street connectivity, density, immigrant concentration, and residential stability."[38]

The results were intriguing. Women living in stable neighborhoods were more likely to be obese, a finding which is not readily explained. But older women living in areas with higher street connectivity were less likely to be overweight or obese. Among men, it was found paradoxically that despite the lower chances of being obese among those who were foreign born, living in areas with higher concentrations of immigrants was linked to higher risk of obesity. Higher income, as expected, meant less obesity.

The authors of the study suggest that these areas should be targeted for interventions: few households of high socioeconomic status, high immigrant concentration, low street connectivity, and high residential stability and older adults.

An analysis of 169 articles published in a 2012 issue of *American Journal of Public Health* found that nearly 90 percent found a "beneficial relationship" between the built environment and physical activity and obesity rates. The catch? Most were observational and failed to prove causality.[39]

Obviously, healthy doses of economics and sociology as well as psychology will be needed to sort out the ideal built environment to fight the obesity epidemic.

SOLUTIONS

People are frustrated by development that requires them to drive long distances between jobs and homes. They are fighting back. Many communities are challenging zoning laws that make it impossible to put workplaces, homes, and services closer together. Others are questioning government decisions that neglect existing infrastructure while expanding new sewers, roads, and services into the suburbs. And still others may be moving back to cities. In *The End of the Suburbs: Where the American Dream is Moving*, Leigh Gallagher writes that American cities are now growing at a faster rate than their suburbs for the first time in 90 years.[40]

Growth can be smart. Growth doesn't need to be a haphazard collage of subdivisions plopped in the middle of farmland and deserts, a deal that steals resources from cities and breeds segregation among people. Communities around the world are seeing that growth doesn't need to lead to sprawl but represents a tremendous opportunity for progress.

Back in 1996, the EPA joined with several nonprofit and government organizations to form the Smart Growth Network (SGN). The network's partners include environmental groups, historic preservation organizations, professional organizations, developers, real estate interests and local and state government entities.

These Smart Growth principles are taken from www.smartgrowth.org:

- *Mixed Land Uses*: Advances in waste management have changed the need for separate zoning for residential, commercial, and industrial uses.

- *Take Advantage of Compact Building Design*: Taxpayers pay less for roads, water, and sewer lines.

- *Create a Range of Housing Opportunities and Choices*: Quality housing should be available for all income levels and age groups as well as less preference for single-family units.

- *Create Walkable Neighborhoods*: Make communities desirable places to live, work, learn, worship, and play.

- *Foster Distinctive, Attractive Communities with a Strong Sense of Place*: Communities should set standards development based on values.

- *Preserve Open Space, Farmland, Natural Beauty, and Critical Environmental Areas*

- *Strengthen and Direct Development Towards Existing Communities*: Direct development toward existing communities already served by infrastructure.

- *Provide a Variety of Transportation Choices* This is key to smart growth.

- *Make Development Decisions Predictable, Fair, and Cost Effective*: Enlist the private sector.

- *Encourage Community and Stakeholder Collaboration*[41]

According to an EPA publication, "growth is smart when it gives us great communities, with more choices and personal freedom, good return on public investment, greater opportunity across the community, a thriving natural environment, and a legacy we can be proud to leave our children and grandchildren."[42]

It's no secret that too many children are obese, a heritage of which we should be ashamed. Fortunately, many new initiatives of governmental and nongovernmental organizations exist to reverse the epidemic. Michelle Obama's mission as First Lady of the United States is to get children more active and eating more nutritiously. Other programs include the CDC's Kids Walk-to-School Campaign; the National Institutes of Health's Ways to Enhance Children's Activity & Nutrition Campaign and Robert Wood Johnson Foundation's Childhood Obesity Initiative. Countries around the world are funding projects in the fight against obesity.

These public health efforts to change behavior are promising.

In 2013, the CDC reported that obesity rates fell slightly in some low-income children in the United States.[43] New policies and programs may be the reason, just as in tobacco control, where public health policies have lowered smoking levels more than individual interventions.[44] Factors such as well-maintained walking surfaces, residential density, public transport, public open space, and mixed land use are important for more walking for recreation and transport.[45] Indeed neighborhoods with "higher walkability scores are associated with significantly more walking."[46]

Exciting new evidence shows that changes in the built environment will affect behavior. A Harvard study reported that "environmental changes in a San Diego naval air station were associated with improvements in the fitness of active-duty personnel, while improved lighting on three urban London streets, and improved bicycle paths on six streets in Toronto were associated with more persons walking and greater bicycle traffic."[47]

Arriving at the main train station in Amsterdam, one sees a

gleaming mass of bicycles parked in a double-decker parking garage. The undisputed leader in encouraging bicycle use among its citizens, the Netherlands offers bike trails and paths in all of its cities. To sweeten the pot, bicyclists have right-of-way advantages at some traffic lights and corners. As a result, 30 percent of all trips made there are by bicycle; compare this to England at 8 percent and the United States at a mere 1 percent.[48] The bicycle, originally called a velocipede, was invented by German Baron Karl von Drais and stands as one of the great inventions of the nineteenth century.[49] It was sought as an alternative to horses. A bicycle, unlike the equine mode of transport, costs little to buy, eats nothing, emits no noxious fumes, takes up little barn space, and requires that a rider burns calories. But the creation that changed the world, the automobile, proved that progress wrapped in tons of steel can inflict major damage. A staggering number in people—over one million—die every year in road traffic crashes around the world. Up to 50 million more suffer nonfatal injuries, according to World Health Organization data. Many of these are young people.[50] Cars are expensive, pollute the air, increase congestion on roadways and parking lots, change the climate, use fossil fuels over which wars are fought and isolate people from their communities. And that's not all. By requiring minimal human energy to operate and by speeding its inhabitants to fast-food windows, automobiles contribute to the obesity epidemic.

So don't wait for the government to step up. Individual choices can also effectively challenge sprawl and its unhealthful effects. While you can't always choose where you work, you can often decide where to live. Make a healthful environment more important than a spacious foyer. This means prioritizing factors that encourage exercise including bike paths, public transport, sidewalks and streets that lead to destinations. This also means changing ideas about exercise. Functional fitness is a popular term describing exercise that accomplishes more than just wearing out running shoes on a treadmill. Walk to the grocery store, even if it is a mile and a half. Too much to carry? Buy less. Bike to church. Too dressed up? Use a city bike and wear flats and change there.

People come up with many reasons not to walk or ride a bike, including bad weather and time limits. Whereas storms and schedules can be valid excuses, most are navigable. Berlin is a model for the rest of the world in this regard. Rain and gray skies are typical there much of the year, but Berliners gamely throw on plastic ponchos and pedal off. And they go at high speeds, thanks to large wheel diameters and unfettered bike paths leading in all directions. In some cases, biking is faster than driving or taking public transport. And Berliners bike to work, school, shops, and even to clubs and parties, because of mandated security measures including well-lit roads and large lamps on bikes. Biking is a way of life supported by citizens and the government. While living in Berlin, I was impressed by the reverence afforded to the bike lane, which is often part of the sidewalk. The hierarchy there has shifted to make bicyclists, not car drivers or pedestrians, the kings of the road, thanks to critical mass.

The final way to challenge sprawl is this: get involved in community initiatives, such as the Smart Growth described above. If your development or town has no such committee or awareness, offer to help organize one. And if that doesn't work, vote with your feet—move to a better place, one that encourages exercise.

5

. . . .

THE FEAR FACTOR: CRIME & OBESITY

Crime is a powerful deterrent to biking to work,
walking home from school, and most activity done outdoors.
And abuse at home can cause obesity too.

WHEN I LEARNED I MAY BE MOVING TO KENYA, one of my first thoughts was of crime. Its glorious flora and fauna aside, a country whose capital is nicknamed the unfortunate "Nai-robbery" is probably not without its security issues. Also bizarrely crossing my mind was that I would gain weight in Nairobi, and not because the food in Kenya would be more delicious or fattening than the *fuul* and *tamiyah* that I had been eating in Egypt. No, it would be because physical activity could be severely limited. I had experienced this before: during the January 25 revolution in Egypt, all residents were under curfew for a few weeks. The government wanted to protect its citizens as well as control them. I had to be back home behind barricaded doors by three o'clock in the afternoon. Outside were looters, thugs, and thousands of escaped prisoners. Even my usual running spot, Wadi Degla canyon, carved from the Pleistocene era hundreds of thousands of years ago, was barred. Gyms were padlocked and school tracks were off limits. Walking anywhere was discouraged, but residents didn't have many places to go unless Tahrir Square with its marauding camels and sundry beasts, most of the human persuasion, was your idea of adventure. So it was sit-ups and push-ups under house arrest for me. Obviously fitness was frivolous when Egyptians were protesting for basic human rights. Still, I craved my basic need to work out. Unhealthy lifestyles also came with the fall of Sadam Hussein and its violent aftermath in Iraq. Wrote *Los Angeles Times* reporter Tina Susman in 2008: "Most retreated to the safety of their homes and became increasingly sedentary, rarely venturing out of their neighborhoods. To go out was to risk being kidnapped, killed by a bomb or caught up in the other violence plaguing Iraq. Curfews hindered people who tried to remain active."[1]

Crime or its potent twin, fear of crime, clearly does not pay in matters of health. Danger in the neighborhood as well as abuse and neglect inside the home are disturbing contributors to the obesity epidemic.

MEAN STREETS

Gang members trading gunfire, punks throwing punches, and drug dealers hanging on street corners—these are familiar scenes for many in poor and immigrant neighborhoods in urban America.

Researchers at the University of Pennsylvania in West Philadelphia work in just such a place; their world-class laboratories and hospitals are surrounded by some of the poorest and most dangerous city blocks in the country. And when the residents of these mean streets venture outside, one thing is obvious: most are overweight or obese. Not too long ago, the Penn scientists set out to see if this observation would hold true in other large cities across the United States. They wondered if mothers of young children would be more obese if they lived in neighborhoods that the women perceived as unsafe. A large sample was taken from the Fragile Families and Child Wellbeing Study, an ambitious project that tracked nearly 5,000 children and their parents spread across 20 cities. Women were asked how often they saw events of social disorder such as loitering adults, gang activity, or drug dealers. The results were clear: women in neighborhoods deemed less safe were more likely to be obese. This held true even after other factors such as household income, education, race, age, marital status, smoking, depression, and television time were controlled.[2]

If people do not feel safe in their neighborhoods, they build walls—both emotional and physical—which can lead to weight gain.

The first wall is fear. Being afraid is a chronic stress. And this type of never-ending stress can lead to obesity. Another chapter deals with this in more detail but here is a short summary: Stress causes release of hormones called glucocorticoids, which lead to weight gain and fat buildup in the abdomen. Meanwhile, in a double whammy, stress stimulates appetite, especially for the so-called "comfort foods," which are foods high in sugar and fat. Foods such as ice cream and french fries calm us down. Comfort foods prompt a sophisticated feedback loop, which in turn elicits a drop in cortisol. This dampens stress and anxiety.[3]

The second wall is made of concrete or brick. If people do not feel safe outdoors, they will spend more time indoors. And because many homes in high-crime areas are not large, this confinement leads to less movement. While experts agree that neighborhood safety can be linked to obesity in several ways, the one most often proposed is crime's blow to physical activity. As we shall see, perception of crime in a neighborhood has an impact on physical exercise across ethnic and age groups. And less physical activity leads to obesity.

Only recently have researchers drawn a firmer line between crime and obesity. One data muddler in the United States was this: while obesity rates had soared in the new millennium, per capita crime had fallen. But as it turned out, this was not true in all communities. The poor and the immigrant populations are heavier, and they live with more crime. For the children in these groups, physical inactivity and obesity are epidemic.

For example, one study probed parents in different neighborhoods about their safety concerns. A questionnaire was given to parents with children in a poor inner-city family practice and to those in a pediatric practice in middle class suburbs. Parents revealed their levels of anxiety concerning gangs, child aggression, crime, traffic, and personal safety in their neighborhood. They also indicated their children's activities.

Unsurprisingly, the inner-city parents expressed much greater anxiety about neighborhood safety than suburban parents. And the inner-city children were less active than these suburban children.[4]

But rural areas also contend with crime. And residents in these areas also say fear keeps them indoors. In 2003, researchers at the School of Public Health at St. Louis University in Missouri telephoned a cross-section of residents living in rural areas of Missouri, Tennessee, and Arkansas; "2,210 respondents were included in the analysis (74% female, 93% white, and 27% obese). The 106-item survey measured perceptions of the neighborhood environment (recreational facilities, land use, transportation/safety, aesthetics, and food environment) and health-related behaviors." After controlling for age, gender, and education, obesity could be linked to several things including distance to recreation facilities and "feeling unsafe from crime."[5] Perception of crime may be just as fattening as crime itself. In other words, behavior and stress follow belief rather than reality.

And what about reactions to actual crime? In the southern United States, in pretty San Antonio, Texas, researchers asked whether adolescents' outdoor physical activity was impacted by violent crime densities.

Environmental factors included the density of violent crime within one-half mile of each participant's home, distance to nearest open play space, per capita income, and a participant's subjective assessment of neighborhood safety. The first, pertaining to density, was linked with girls' outdoor activity. And if girls thought the neighborhood was safe, they played more outdoors. The boys were different: thoughts on safety down their block did not relate to the amount of time spent in outdoor play.

The conclusion was that "neighborhood violent crime may be a significant environmental barrier to outdoor physical activity for urban dwelling Mexican-American adolescent girls."[6]

The opposite of physical activity is sedentary activity, oxymoronic as it may sound. Another study done in Texas related indoor sedentary behavior with community crime statistics. While some of this will be discussed in the chapter on sleep, it is interesting in what it says about how modern parents protect their families in the face of unsafe neighborhoods or the perception of unsafe neighborhoods.[7]

The authors write: "Over the past 30 years, technological changes have made the indoor alternatives to playing outside, where children are more vulnerable to criminal activity, more enjoyable (cable TV, video games, and the Internet) and comfortable (the spread of air-conditioning to low income neighborhoods)."[8]

The study looked at fourth-graders, approximately an even number of girls and boys; nearly half of the group was Hispanic. Boys spent 5.2 hours a day in sedentary behaviors with television, computers, and video games. Girls spent much less time with Xbox and PlayStation, and, as a result, their average sedentary time was lower at 3.6 hours a day. Crime statistics in the city of the school were charted: sexual offenders per capita, robberies, all violent crimes, murders, assaults, property crimes, rapes, burglaries, larcenies, and motor vehicle thefts.

The results were intriguing. Boys spent more time with video games when their community had more sex offenders and burglaries. A mere percentage point increase in per capita sex offenders translated into an increase of 1.7 hours of video game playing per day. Burglaries had a much smaller effect: a larger 10-percent increase would only add 2 minutes and 40 seconds to the sessions. Girls living in a sea of sexual predators reacted differently than the boys. They went on the computer less: a percentage point increase in sexual predators was associated with less computer time—48 minutes less per day. The authors suspected that "parents in these communities may be reluctant to allow their girls to be potentially exposed to online sexual advances." Moreover, under Texas law, crime of sexual predation can be announced through the mail, advertisements, and the Internet. It is possible, the authors thought, that the exposure and thus fear of this sort of crime is more prevalent than to those less publicized.[9]

Another development is that as more children use inside leisure technologies, fewer friends are outdoors. The wisdom of "safety in numbers" may force more children indoors, as they see fewer peers outside.

My childhood home in Pennsylvania lies across the street from an elementary school. The attached playground was the joy of my summers: volleyball, basketball, crafts, hopscotch, dancing, baseball, kickball, water-balloon battles, biking, and picnics. I returned to the old neighborhood often when my children were young. During early visits, I was not surprised to see basketball nets dangling in shreds; after all, tall young players often get rambunctious. But then one summer, the metal rims were missing, either yanked or severed from the backboards. The final blow came later when a massive trailer with additional classrooms was parked in the middle of the basketball court. Other summers saw my son being harassed by teens and young men when he rode his bike or ventured out to other basketball courts. Video games and television soon became more appealing to this active kid. Undeniably, jungle gyms, baseball fields, and bike lanes are not the answer if people are too frightened to go out and use them.

Many young people across the globe are not meeting the recommended levels for exercise. Researchers in North Carolina asked the question directly: what stood in the way of physical activity? "Thirteen focus groups were conducted with 41 young people and 50 parents from [the eastern part of the state]." Their answers? Crime and danger stood out as barriers along with other factors including distance and cost.[10] And on the flip side, fifth-graders in Nova Scotia were surveyed, and researchers found that children in safe neighborhoods engaged more in unsupervised sports.[11]

African-American populations suffer from higher rates of obesity than the general population. In the United States in 2009, half of all adult black females were obese, as opposed to one-third of white women, according to the CDC. Conjectures for these differences range from socioeconomic differences to attitudes to genes. But one factor is evident. More African-Americans cluster in inner city urban areas where crime can be higher.

In 2009, researchers at Johns Hopkins Bloomberg School of Public Health in Baltimore, Maryland, conducted a literature search focused on African-Americans to explore this vein. Results? Sidewalks and safety from crime translated into more physical activity.[12]

It is true that not all studies point to a link. For instance, one study asked if safety of children's neighborhoods (as well as proximity to playgrounds and to fast-food restaurants) would impact weight status of preschoolers.[13] The setting was Cincinnati, Ohio, a city in the midwestern part of the United States. The participants were more than 7,000 low-income children between three and six years old. Neighborhood safety was defined by the number of police-reported crimes per 1,000 residents per year in each of 46 city neighborhoods. Overall, 9.2 percent of the children were overweight, 76 percent black, and 23 percent white. No association was found between child overweight and proximity to playgrounds, proximity to fast-food restaurants, or level of neighborhood crime. Other studies fail to make the case that crime impacts physical activity. But some obesity researchers suspect that research methods may be the problem. Gary G. Bennett and colleagues in the exhaustive *Obesity Epidemiology* text argue that there is considerable variation in measuring crime and safety in much of the research on this subject. In addition, they wrote, "few of the studies in this area have directly examined obesity outcomes despite the clear potential for perceived neighborhood safety to increase obesity risk, particularly among those in low-income and urban environments."[14]

Crime data are confusing. Even something as straightforward as homicide numbers can be fudged by semantics, cover-ups, or poor record keeping. Nevertheless, a 2011 study undertaken by the Geneva Declaration on Armed Violence and Development estimated that at least 526,000 people worldwide die violently every year, more than three-quarters of them in non-conflict settings. One-quarter of all violent deaths occur in just 14 countries, seven of which are in the Americas. Although wars dominate media headlines, the levels of armed violence in some non-conflict countries resemble those of conflict zones. In an average year between 2004 and 2009, more people per capita were killed in El Salvador than in Iraq.

Take a look at these numbers for homicides per 100,000 people, published by the United Nations Office on Drugs and Crime in 2012:[15]

- Japan (.4)
- Germany (.8)
- Egypt (1.2)
- United States (4.2)
- Russian Federation (10.2)
- Honduras (91.6)

The United States falls in the middle when you look at international statistics. But if you live in a place called Oakland, California, your chances of getting killed are higher than many other places.

A group of 359 adults who lived in that city were surveyed on walking habits and matched up against crime data from the Oakland Police Department. Not surprisingly, the higher the violent crime rate, the less walking was done.[16]

The fact that murder can be peacefully low in a place like Japan (which also boasts one of the world's lowest obesity rates at 3%) but perilously high in Honduras proves that humanity is capable of more.

New York City has done a remarkable job of decreasing crime on their streets. Many credit targeted police policies for their success. With its colorful quilt of residential homes, businesses, schools, hospitals, and parks, the city provides a perfect living laboratory for Columbia University researchers to study obesity and the environment in their own backyard. While research confirms that easy access to parks means more exercise, they flipped the question: what would deter exercise in the parks? "Crime, pedestrian safety, and noxious land uses" all dissuade residents from enjoying their parks and playgrounds. The authors suggest that safe and pleasant passage to the park may be just as important as having a park in some neighborhoods.[17] Improving neighborhood safety is a "promising strategy" to reduce obesity.[18]

A community in South Carolina is moving in that direction. Researchers at the University of South Carolina have designed a trial to increase walking in low income, ethnic minority communities. The Positive Action for Today's Health (PATH) trial is comparing three communities randomly assigned to different interventions to improve safety and access for walking. One group has police-patrolled walking plus social marketing, another police-patrolled-walking only, and the last, a general health intervention. The results should be interesting.[19]

Times have changed. Doors stay locked. Sex offender alerts keep children inside. Children are supervised every minute of every day. We may need to accept that.

But many experts feel policy makers need to be more proactive.

Authors of the Texas study concluded that "children still likely prefer to socialize, play team sports, and to roam free outdoors. Therefore, after-school programs promoting physical activity which feature adult supervision should be expanded because they will ease parental fears about crime. Team sports, which in years past would form spontaneously, must be organized by parents."[20]

Unfortunately, many physical education programs have been cut along with athletic teams at many school districts hardest hit by finance troubles.

Because crime will not disappear overnight, communities must make these important policy choices today, so as not to doom the present generation to poor health.

In addition to civic action, individuals must step up. Besides being good role models, parents must make exercise a priority for their family, as important as homework, music lessons, and sharing the day's events at dinner.

DANGER AT HOME

Sadly, home is not always a sanctuary. Sexual abuse, verbal cruelty, beatings, and neglect occur daily in millions of homes across the world. The fallout from such abuse is wide: self-mutilation, mood disorders, drug addiction, and alcoholism. And, as it turns out, obesity.

More and more, research indicates that childhood abuse of many kinds is associated with excess body weight later in life.

One way to study this is to go to very obese people and ask them about their childhoods. Not surprisingly, the heaviest people often carried the saddest baggage. For example, the Adverse Childhood Experiences Study, which surveyed more than 13,000 members of a California health maintenance organization, found that a history of abuse was more likely in those with BMI ≥40 than to those with BMI ≥30.[21] More than a decade earlier in 1991, another California study reported higher rates of morbid obesity (>100 pounds overweight) among individuals with a history of childhood sexual abuse.[22]

Many morbidly obese people undergo surgery by which key parts of the gut are either restricted or rerouted. More than 160,000 of these bariatric procedures are performed each year in the United States alone.

Does this group report more childhood abuse?

A 2006 study headed by Thomas Wadden at the University of Pennsylvania compared extremely obese women about to undergo bariatric surgery to women with lesser obesity who were enrolled in a behavioral weight loss program. The bariatric group revealed higher rates of childhood physical and sexual abuse.[23] About the same time, a team at Yale asked 340 extremely obese candidates for gastric bypass surgery to complete a questionnaire measuring childhood trauma. Nearly 70 percent reported childhood maltreatment.[24] Similar numbers were reported in bariatric candidates at the University of Pittsburgh.[25]

Before there was gastric bypass, morbidly obese people tried, among many other things, very-low-calorie diets. In the early 1990s, one hundred enrollees in just such a regimen in Southern California were interviewed. "By comparison with a control group of 100 always-slender adults, the obese applicants were found to be [quite] different." They were much more likely to have experienced "childhood sexual abuse, nonsexual childhood abuse, early parental loss, parental alcoholism, chronic depression, and marital family dysfunction in their own adult lives."[26]

Scattered studies show that childhood abuse can lead to obesity in adulthood. Most research on the topic is centered in large medical centers in the United States, presumably because the country is home to many obese people. But other countries, with obesity rates not far behind, are asking similar questions.

In the United Kingdom, at the Institute of Child Health Study at University College London, researchers looked at over 9,000 individuals all of whom were born during one week in March 1958 in England, Scotland, and Wales. They were interviewed in childhood (ages 7, 11, and 16 years) and adulthood (23, 33, 42, and 45 years). "The risk of obesity increased by 20% to 50% for several adversities (physical abuse, verbal abuse, witnessed abuse, humiliation, neglect, strict upbringing, physical punishment, conflict or tension, low parental aspirations or interest in education, [few] outings with parents, and father hardly reads to child)."[27]

In Australia, from surveys at the University of Queensland, the prevalence of overweight and obesity at age 21 was greater in young women who suffered penetrative sexual abuse before age sixteen. "Of [the] 1,305 women [polled], 20.6% reported non-penetrative and 7.9% reported penetrative [sexual abuse] by age 16." Non-penetrative sexual abuse in women was not linked. In a group of nearly 1,300 men surveyed, neither type of sexual abuse was associated with overweight.[28]

In one group of obese girls in an Israeli clinic, those abused were more obese. All of the maltreated girls had other changes including "seductive behavior, seclusion, self-mutilation, and new onset day enuresis."[29]

Girls in particular appear to be at high risk for obesity long after abuse. One study tracked the same girls over a 20-year span, in what is called a longitudinal study. From ages 6 to 20, obesity rates in 84 abused girls were not different from their non-abused counterparts. But by young adulthood (ages 20–27), the abused females were more likely to be obese (42%) than the others (28%).[30]

The gap widens as women age. By middle age, those who had been victimized by physical or sexual abuse were twice as likely to be obese than non-abused women. This result was determined by questioning nearly 5,000 women enrolled in a health insurance plan. "A telephone survey assessed child sexual and physical abuse, obesity, . . . depressive symptoms, binge eating, and body dissatisfaction."[31]

To a lesser extent, boys can be vulnerable to weight gain with negative treatment, especially when they grow from adolescence into adulthood. Some data link domestic violence to a risk of unhealthy weight during adolescence in boys.[32]

Parents are a profound environmental influence. Being a good parent is a tightrope walk for any man or woman. The challenges are considerable. Working too much to provide for the family may risk neglect, especially for single parents. Heeding older family members who advise not to spare the rod can escalate into harsh spankings. Caring too much can cross into overindulgence, helicopter parenting, or tiger mothering. What effect, if any, could these nonsexual abuses—neglect, hitting, or threatening the child—have on obesity?

Temple University's Robert C. Whitaker and team mined data from the Fragile Families and Child Wellbeing Study, "the birth cohort study . . . of nearly 5,000 children born between 1998 and 2,000 in 20 large US cities."[33] At three years of age, half had their heights and weights recorded and their mothers answered the Parent-Child Conflict Tactics Scales regarding three types of child maltreatment—neglect, corporal punishment, and psychological aggression. The most prevalent types of corporal punishment were spanking the child on the bottom with a bare hand and slapping the child on the hand, arm, or leg. The two most prevalent types of psychological aggression were shouting, yelling, or screaming at the child and threatening to spank or hit the child but not actually doing it. The design controlled a string of variables: age, income, number of children in the household, the mother's ethnicity, education, marital status, body mass index, prenatal smoking, and the children's sex and birth weight.

The results were surprising. Neither corporal punishment nor psychological aggression was associated with obesity. It was neglect that changed the odds of obesity; nearly 50 percent higher for those participants.

The authors suggested an explanation: the first two are common discipline techniques that parents use in response to their children's misbehavior. And, which is important, a child might come to anticipate the punishment. In contrast, neglect is not usually prompted by the child's misbehavior and may be unpredictable. Possibly, they add, "it may be the unexpected or non-contingent nature of neglect that heightens the child's emotional distress." Or maybe the toddlers most likely to merit discipline are the ones most active and least likely to be overweight.

The underlying mechanisms by which child maltreatment may lead to later obesity are uncertain, as we shall see in the next section. But there are likely to be many.

How Abuse Leads to Obesity

Abused or neglected children cope in several ways. Because the abuser is a family member or visitor to their home, the child feels helpless to escape the situation. So the trapped child adapts in other ways, some by choice and others of which they may not be aware: they may gain weight on purpose; eat comfort foods; increase stress hormones; increase anger vigilance; disrupt reproductive hormones. All of these can lead to weight gain.

Adaptations to abuse:

- Intentional weight gain: Some who have been abused sexually will purposefully gain weight to discourage attacks. "Obese patients [in one study] commonly reported using obesity as a sexually protective device; many reported overeating to cope with emotional distress."[34]

- Comfort foods: Eating comfort foods will make them feel better. And as is explained in the chapter on stress, it is not because ice cream and cake feel like happy foods. No, high-fat and sugary foods physically tamp down the body's stress response. This sort of emotion-focused coping is often employed to reduce distress when the stressor itself cannot be eliminated.[35]

- Brain and hormonal changes: Chronic stress caused by abuse can literally change the brain. It can change how the brain drives the engine of energy. This takes place along a sophisticated highway called the hypothalamic-pituitary-adrenal (HPA) axis. Changes in the HPA axis and surges in cortisol and insulin can lead to poor appetite control. Stress encourages new fat cells and directs them toward places such as the stomach. In addition, MRI studies have revealed differences in other parts of the brain, including the corpus callosum, hippocampus, and amygdala. Disconcertingly, changes in gene expression and behavior that encourages obesity may be transmitted across generations, stamping a biological birthmark even on those never exposed to mistreatment.[36]

- Heightened defensive emotions: If you have ever watched daytime television with Jerry Springer or his ilk, you will see some very angry people. They have to be paid actors, you think; no one gets that vitriolic. But possibly they are betraying earlier abuse. Maltreated children may experience more negative emotions, specifically anger, fear, and aggression. In addition, they are hypervigilant or on guard to outside threats. Over time, these frequent expressions of anger may have a toxic effect on fat tissue.[37] Anger can encourage buildup of central fat, the most dangerous kind, in both adults[38] and in adolescents.[39]

- Reproductive hormones change: During puberty, "abused [and] neglected children have disrupted regulation of reproductive hormones," which impact fat levels during midlife and menopause.[40]

Children aren't the only household members who are abused. Women and men of all ages are physically and verbally abused or neglected. Many of the above mechanisms also apply to adults. Much of the research, however, has centered on child abuse and its associations with obesity. But in another troubling outcome, women who are victims of chronic intimate partner violence have been shown to have heavier preschool children.

How Much Abuse?

In many countries, before the gentler wisdom of pediatrician Benjamin Spock held sway, corporal punishment or physical penalty was routine. Children were to "be seen and not heard" and therefore suffered more abuse in silence. Many children lived with sexual, physical, and verbal abuse, and neglect. Today, we like to think we are more enlightened regarding child rearing (until the next generation of theories). In many families, children are anything but neglected: they are the center of the parents' universe and share family resources with few siblings. Yet the modern world and its social changes bring many potential occasions for child abuse. There are more divorces and remarriages today, leaving blended families in which young children and teens live with stepparents and stepsiblings, entirely unrelated by blood. Temptation and intolerance may be more likely in such situations. Also, many more single mothers are having children, though the number has stabilized in some countries. Unattached women may bring boyfriends and other unrelated males into the home, exposing children to possible abuse. In addition, a single parent's strain of raising young children is not softened by sharing the burden with a spouse. And finally, in a western culture of heightened sexuality and violence in movies and video games, the propensity for such behavior is likely increased.

A history of childhood sexual abuse is not uncommon; it may affect up to one in three women and one out of eight men.[41]

And given that child protection services agencies continue to investigate cases of maltreatment involving millions of children each year, this crime may be an important contributor to the obesity epidemic.

Abuse may be even more of an obesogenic factor in the developing world, a place where women and children can be revered but just as often are considered chattel. Beatings and sexual abuse can be common but statistics are less reliable. Making matters worse is that the abused may have few places to turn because of a society that either accepts abuse or turns a blind eye to it. Resorting to coping mechanisms and physical adaptations that encourage obesity are likely.

SOLUTIONS

When violence inside the home leads to obesity later in life, it may appear that the damage is done. But there are two ideas that may be helpful.

First, when child welfare therapists or caseworkers handle situations with abused children, in addition to eliminating the abuser, they should be mindful of dysfunctional coping mechanisms that may lead to obesity. Referral to a dietitian or a psychologist may prevent later problems.[42] New obesity prevention strategies, ones that begin very early in life, include efforts not solely focused on diet and activity and may prevent more than obesity.[43]

And second, nutrition practitioners can help obese patients recognize how they got that way. If abuse is a part of that story then referral to child welfare or therapists may interrupt the sad cycle.

Because danger inside and outside the home can lead to obesity, fighting crime will help in fighting fat.

Health is too valuable to surrender lightly.

6

. . . .

DRIVE-BY FEEDINGS: TOXIC FOOD LANDSCAPE & OBESITY

Instant gratification paired with assault marketing will undo the best of intentions.

SOMETHING'S HAPPENING IN EGYPT THAT HAS nothing to do with overthrowing a government and everything to do with revolting new trends in fast food.

Shops selling sweet confections are taking over my neighborhood of Maadi, a leafy outpost just below Cairo. Auntie Loulou's offers waffle and crepes, and a place called Pumpkin features gooey tarts and pies. Nearby ChaCho sells more waffles. Maadi has a Marriott hotel bakery, a French dessert shop, and even an Auntie Anne's.

Yes, this familiar pretzel franchise has opened here on Road 9, a dusty potholed bazaar and a far cry from the air-conditioned malls of suburban America. One of their signature products, a pretzel dressed up as a doughnut, is a hit. And in a nod to the Middle East, the Auntie Anne's menu in Maadi offers a Kofta Pretzel Combo: a spicy mini-meatloaf sheathed in a soft pretzel paired with soda and fried potato wedges. A bargain, perhaps, at 20 Egyptian pounds (US $3) but no treat for the arteries.

You can play a game with these menus. What to choose if forced to order something nutritious, or at the very least, an item not considered unhealthy? Hmm. Among the meat pretzels, sweet pretzels, chocolate dips, milkshakes, and syrupy lemonades, this Auntie Anne's sells water, not the chain's attempt at nutrition, a honey whole-grain pretzel. Tea or coffee would be acceptable too. (According to the website, if you want your pretzel without butter or salt, they will accommodate you).

And then just when I thought my nutrition radar couldn't take any more fatty and sugary temptations so close to home, the cupcake invasion hit Cairo. Crumbs Cupcakes & More had come to hard-scrabble Road 9, obviously an avenue with identity issues. Gourmet cupcakes are so profitable in the United States that one company publicly trades on the NASDAQ exchange. Soon after, in inscrutable Egyptian style, other cupcake shops moved in steps away.

Cinnabon tried to get a foothold on the same street but failed. When many foreigners moved on during the revolution, so did this usually successful chain known for its gargantuan-sized pastries. I wasn't unhappy. Egyptians already have enough sweet temptations in the form of traditional dishes like *basbousa*, a semolina cake soaked in syrup and *om' ali*, a rich nutty pudding. A wildly popular bakery nearby called Koueider has been selling these and more for decades.

It is no secret that Egyptians are putting on pounds. In 2010, 76 percent of women were overweight and 48 percent were obese.[1] It comes as no surprise then that diabetes is skyrocketing in Egypt and all across the region; seven of the ten countries with the highest prevalence for diabetes are in the Middle East. Do they really need another loaded gun from the American arsenal of fast-food chains?

TASTY, CHEAP, AND EASY

Modern life is making the world obese. The World Health Organization reports that more people are obese than undernourished. Look at the latest numbers: nearly 1.5 billion overweight and over one-half billion obese. In some countries, more than one in four children is overweight. Obesity has doubled in the last several decades in the majority of high-income countries. And sadly, most other countries including the poorest have followed close behind.[2]

How did this happen? Human biology has not changed in the last twenty years. Our environment, however, has changed dramatically. We now have an obesogenic environment.

"Obesity is the result of people responding normally to the

obesogenic environments they find themselves in." This conclusion is from global obesity researchers who authored a seminal paper published in an August 2011 issue of the journal *Lancet*.[3] It is a radical reversal: it is not just lack of will power making people obese.

What exactly is this obesogenic environment? Is it the fast-food temptations on every corner? Is it brilliant food marketing? Or perhaps it is simple economics: does healthy food cost too much? As we will see, it is all of these and more.

History of nourishment in a nutshell: Humans swung from trees as hunter-gatherers, stalking meat and foraging for seeds, berries, and leaves. All of their energy went into these tasks. Much later, agriculture was born. A plot of land would yield plenty of food, at least some years in some places. Most of their energy went into these tasks. And then, fast-forward to the late 1800s—the industrial complex, with its giant strides in efficiency and specialization transformed food production. Not only was it cheaper but also more of it was available all the time. As a result, very little, if any, energy goes into putting food in our mouths these days. In addition, bringing us to the key message in this chapter, modern food has loads of fat and calories. Energy balance is thrown off-kilter, hardly a paean to progress.

New York University nutrition professor Marion Nestle writes in her important book *Food Politics*: "Also ironic is that once people become better off, they are observed to enter a 'nutrition transition' in which they abandon traditional plant-based diets and begin eating more meat, fat, and processed foods. The result is a sharp increase in obesity and related chronic diseases."[4]

Nestle adds that "humans do not innately know how to select a nutritious diet . . ."[5] This is an incredible statement and an acquittal of sorts for obese people. Of course, humans will sense specific survival needs, such as sugar in hypoglycemia and water in dehydration as well as a condition called pica in which dirt and paint chips are eaten for mineral value. But as for the rest of the menu, humans are simply confused. And if the menu selections are vast and affordable—and it has never been more so than today—choosing really gets muddled. Need versus want is the perpetual challenge.

"When food is plentiful and people can afford to buy it, basic biological needs become less compelling and the principal determinant of food choice is personal preference," writes Nestle.[6]

And what do humans prefer? Three words: tasty, cheap, and easy.

Tasty: humans favor sugar and fat; seeking calorie-dense foods is hardwired into our taste buds. An early hominid who preferred weeds to a fresh carcass most likely did not survive.

Cheap: ingredients in items such as potato chips and soda cost little, giving manufacturers huge incentives to flood the market with processed junk foods. The competition drives down prices in the snack aisle, where a mega-size bag of chips can be more affordable than a sack of potatoes. And thanks to high-fructose corn syrup (HFCS), sodas are always cheaper than milk and juices. The United States government controls food prices through a bounty of tricks: price supports, production quotas, import restrictions, favorable tax rates, and inexpensive land leases are just a few. Some of these policies push up energy intake. Also, when income inequality rises, so does obesity.[7]

Easy: Societies have changed. Women in many countries work outside the home. Women are no longer able to spend time shopping, cooking, or cleaning up. Yet a typical middle-class kitchen has a stove, oven, dishwasher, garbage disposal, refrigerator, and freezer, as well as a counter topped with a toaster, blender, food processor, microwave, toaster oven, coffee maker, one-cup coffee maker, cappuccino maker, mixer, and more stored in the cupboard: coffee grinder, yogurt maker, ice cream freezer, bread maker, pasta maker, waffle maker, pancake grill, hamburger maker, beer brewer, meat slicer, deep fryer, meat smoker, and, way in the back, a beef jerky apparatus. People with more money buy computerized refrigerators, stand-alone freezers, and grill top stoves with eight burners. The modern family kitchen is better equipped than most restaurants in New York City.

As the number of machines has gone up, time spent in the kitchen has gone down. The microwave alone spawned entire supermarket aisles and deep freezers of convenience foods, ensuring that people exert fewer calories preparing food.

Profound changes in the food environment have occurred in the past few decades. Let's use the United States as an example because it is a country with plenty of statistics.

- The share of daily calories from food eaten away from home went from 18 percent to 32 percent between the late 1970s and the middle 1990s, according to the USDA's food-intake surveys.[8]

- 42 percent of the food dollar in 2006 was for food consumed away from home.[9]

- About half of restaurant meals are now from fast-food restaurants.[10]

"Societal changes easily explain why nearly half of all meals are consumed outside the home, a quarter of them as fast food, and that the practice of snacking nearly doubled from the mid-1980s to the mid-1990s," wrote Nestle.[11]

Tasty, cheap, and easy is the winning trifecta that has been perfected by the fast-food industry. Since Ray Croc opened his first McDonald's franchise in 1954, the fast-food phenomenon has spread from sea to shining sea and on to every other continent. Fast-food joints piggybacked the highways that crisscrossed the vast miles of twentieth-century America. Now, they are everywhere: gas stations, drugstores, shopping malls, airports, schools, and hospitals.

In 1970, Americans spent about $6 billion on fast food. By 2010, that number rose to an astounding $165 billion.[12]

Fast-food chains are a familiar sight in most corners of the world. McDonald's golden arches greet visitors at the Pyramids, the Eiffel Tower, the Brandenburg Gate, and the Great Wall of China. Hamburger diplomacy fields over 32,000 stores in more than 100 countries. But it took a colonel to enter Kenya.

Kentucky Fried Chicken (KFC) opened in its capital city of Nairobi in 2011. It was the first American brand fast-food franchise to open in all of East Africa. Jason Straziuso of the Associated Press reported that "the restaurant's . . . opening was met with long lines of enthusiastic customers. Some waited up to 90 minutes to be served [fried chicken] . . . The Nairobi KFC investor group includes a man whose family owns 40 KFC restaurants in South Africa . . . The group wants to open 15 restaurants in Kenya, Tanzania and Uganda [by 2014]." Obesity rates in Kenya pale compared to those in South Africa. So far.[13]

South Africans enjoy fast foods from western chains as well as their traditional street foods. In one study, those with higher incomes preferred fast foods and the poor went for street foods. A one-week survey there of street food consumption showed that fresh fruit was the biggest seller and also that blacks purchased more soft drinks and savory snacks than did whites.[14]

Street food—or indie fast-food—can be healthy. Fruit juice stands are too plentiful to count in Cairo. Stroll over and order a tall glass of fresh, unsweetened pomegranate, grapefruit, or mango juice. Then grab a bag of hot peanuts from an outdoor roaster or a charred sweet potato from a donkey cart rigged with an oven no bigger than an Easy-Bake. Other offerings from street stalls, such as deep-fried chickpea fritters called *falafels* or plastic baggies filled with sugar water are less attractive to a nutrition-minded customer. This choice between healthy and junk is seen around the world: *currywurst* in Berlin, hot dogs in Manhattan, and deep-fried bread called *bedmi* in India are not far from the fruit stand, popcorn machine, or pistachio wagon. But all street foods have one healthy advantage over the newer fast-food franchises: you walk up to buy. You expend calories getting there.

Fast-food franchises also run the gamut on the nutrition spectrum. Some offer healthy choices. Auntie Anne's in Maadi did not. McDonald's offers salads with low-calorie dressings and skim milk. Subway's better options include whole wheat bread, tomatoes, and lean turkey slices. Subway, which has surpassed McDonald's in number of shops around the world, enjoyed a public relations coup when a young man named Jared Fogle lost 245 pounds on what was dubbed the Subway Diet. Morgan Spurlock proved the opposite in his book *Don't Eat This Book: Fast Food and the Supersizing of America*: eating breakfast, lunch, and dinner—supersizing when asked— at McDonald's for one month spurred a 24.5-pound weight gain and spikes in his cholesterol and liver enzymes.[15] Publicity stunts? Sure. A person can lose weight eating a McDonald's salad and a hamburger every day or gain weight on double meat and cheese hoagies on wheat buns. The truth as usual lies somewhere in the middle.

Fast foods in general are loaded with calories, fats, and sugars. Fast food is associated with higher body mass index (BMI), weight gain, and less successful weight-loss maintenance.[16] People who eat regularly at fast-food places are more likely to be obese: they had odds of being obese that were 60 to 80 percent higher compared with those people who ate fast food less than once per week. Several studies showed the same.[17]

Take this a step further. Will having a McDonald's down the street make people more likely to visit? Does proximity to fast food increase obesity?

Greater neighborhood fast-food availability is linked, if precariously, to more obesity. Six studies found higher body mass index was associated with living in areas with more fast food; four studies, however, did not.[18] One large study looked at 13,000 young adults and proximity to fast food and their consumption of fast food. When looked at in this manner, instead of in terms of obesity, there was no correlation. It could be, the authors pose, that fast-food outlets favor areas accessible by car, which use itself would encourage obesity.[19]

A unique feature of fast-food sites is the ability to drive up and order food. Sitting in a caravan of exhaust fumes may not appeal to you, but you would be in the minority. Most people love it. Nearly 65 percent of McDonald's menu in the United States is passed out of a tiny window into a waiting car. These rates are surely lower in less car-centric cultures such as Europe. Tom Vanderbilt in *Slate Magazine* online tells of the painstaking design of the drive-thru model, which he learned of in *QSR* or (quick-service restaurant) magazine:

> Wireless headset technology has been credited with increasing traffic by as much as fifty cars an hour at some McDonald's stores. Other time-savers include stochastic queuing models, multilane drive-throughs (a perception-management tool as much as anything else, as research shows visibly longer lines deter would-be drive-through customers), and technologies like "Clear Sound," which "processes all sounds present at the drive-thru lane and eliminates extraneous ambient noises such as idling engines, mufflers and nearby traffic."[20]

Don't try to walk or bike up to a drive-thru, however. Most

companies' policies say you won't be served. Sophisticated improvements to customer service make fast food even faster. Smartphone apps now allow customers to order and pay before you pick up at places like McDonald's and Starbucks. "When you have a very comfortable ordering environment, like a smartphone, you just order more," app maker for Kentucky Fried Chicken Jeremie Leroyer told the *Financial Times* in 2013.[21]

With franchises selling on so many corners, you have to wonder: Could fast food be addicting? Some scientists think so. They see sugar addiction in rodents and point out that many fast food meals come with sugary beverages. Evidence also suggests that the high fat and salt content of fast food may spawn addiction. Caffeine is indisputably addictive and special coffee drinks have proven a hit on fast food menus.[22] While the theory of fast-food addiction remains fluid, any parent will attest that a glimpse of the golden arches triggers a Pavlovian response in children.

Fast food is not the only reason we're getting fatter. Anyone who has ever eaten at Old Country Buffet knows that eating in full-service restaurants, or almost no-service in this case, can be equally fattening. Smorgasbords, buffets, all-you-can-eat, free refills, and the like have never been more popular. For anyone who was taught to eat every last smidgen on her plate, like me, these banquets of overload are dangerous. I clearly remember my first smorgasbord, such a rarity back then; it was destination dining with an exotic flavor. My parents dressed all eight children in church clothes and introduced us to the wonders of novelty and abundance. We were revolted by the tiny frog legs but smitten with the endless scoops of ice cream. Today, there are countless venues for this kind of eating, from all-you-can-eat deep-dish pies at Pizza Hut in London to bountiful Ramadan buffets at Middle Eastern hotels. My most recent, in 2012 at a strip mall in my hometown, offered hundreds of appetizing dishes, literally hundreds—an entire Chinese takeout menu was displayed under heat lamps, from sushi to egg rolls to every variety of chicken, pork, beef, shrimp, and noodle and rice combo. The owners didn't skimp; broiled salmon, clams, mussels, crab, steak, and even pizza and mayonnaise chicken and tuna salads were available if Asian food wasn't your preference. For dessert they offered rows of sweet buns, pastries, cakes, and buckets of ice cream alongside caramel and chocolate toppings. The price of such a cornucopia? $6.25.

Willpower crumbles in face of such variety. Science says so.

Faced with an assortment of foods, studies show, people do eat more. Pennsylvania State University's Barbara Rolls knows all about eating patterns. From her extensive research, Rolls fashioned a weight-management concept based on low calorie-dense foods, which became wildly popular among nutritionists and dieters alike. The first book of three, *Volumetrics Weight-Control Plan*, came out over ten years ago and still sells strongly.[23]

While everyone needs a variety of foods for optimal nutrition, Rolls confirmed that the more types of food available, the more people tend to eat. "What happens during a meal of many different foods or courses is that we experience satiety for each food as we eat it," Rolls said in an interview with *Real Simple* magazine. "But we are still 'hungry' for foods we haven't eaten yet, particularly those that have different tastes, aromas, shapes, textures, and other sensory properties."[24]

Italian, Mexican, French, seafood, steak houses, and other restaurant menus offer endless variety compared to the home kitchen. It follows from Rolls's research that eating out in general—not just at buffets—will increase hunger and appetite. And studies do show that the more often you eat out, the fatter you will be. And along those lines, the more restaurants per capita, the higher the obesity levels.[25]

Eating out then, whether at fast food or full-service, is mined with obesity triggers. Eating at home may be one answer. This takes us to supermarkets, which have their own special confusing place in the obesity puzzle.

FOOD DESERT OR FOOD SWAMP?

Piggly Wiggly opened the first self-service grocery store in the United States in 1916. The name itself portends less than svelte outcomes for customers. According to Spurlock, by 1940 there were almost 3,000 Piggly Wiggly locations nationwide.[26] Safeway, A&P,

King Cullen, Ralph's, Kroger, and the rest followed. With their aisles of products all vying for the shopper's attention, these stores made brand names and packaging important for the first time. By 1955, 60 percent of our food was bought in supermarkets.

Supermarkets pushed out all but the most stubborn mom and pop grocers. The charm of these small shops—tacked onto corners of most streets—belies the fact that they sold lots of junk food. Mrs. Howells waited patiently as we chose penny candy from a glass case filled with a hundred choices. And Nader's basement shop was where, with their paper route money, my twin brothers stopped for soda, a beverage forbidden at home. It wasn't all fruits and vegetables by any means. These were the early versions of 7-Eleven and Wawa convenience stores, without the lottery tickets. Consequently, when supermarkets emerged as clear winners in the retail wars, it was no great loss to our collective nutrition; it was a move into more possibility for better food with its endless variety, convenience, and coupons.

Has it worked out that way? Obesity keeps rising, so you have to wonder if supermarkets are the panacea they promised.

On the one hand, many studies suggest that access to supermarkets is related to healthier food intake and lower levels of obesity because supermarkets may offer a variety of high-quality products at lower cost. Low income and minority communities in the United States tend to suffer from worse access to supermarkets and healthy food choices, at the same time as greater exposure to fast food outlets and convenience stores.[27]

Communities lacking in supermarkets have been labeled "food deserts." These food deserts have been fingered as one cause of obesity, which is more common in disadvantaged zip codes. Studies, initiatives, and government interventions have rallied behind getting healthier food options into these poor communities where "at least 500 people and/or at least 33 percent of the census tract's population must reside more than one mile from a supermarket or more than 10 miles in a rural area."[28] According to the USDA, 2.5 million households[29] in the United States may fit that description. But a study from the Public Policy Institute of California found that the low-income areas in a state survey actually had more retail food vendors of all types (fast food, corner stores, and supermarkets) than wealthier neighborhoods.[30] Further muddying the landscape is the fact that 93 percent of people in low-income, low-access areas do their shopping with a vehicle, according to a USDA report.[31] Nevertheless, even if the food desert concept has some cracks in it, the question remains: will people eat healthier foods if they have a supermarket close by?

New research from the University of North Carolina at Chapel Hill says no. It contradicts earlier data and shows that people didn't eat more fruits and vegetables when they had supermarkets in their neighborhoods. Income and nearby fast-food restaurants influenced choices more. More than 5,000 people over 15 years in four cities took part in the study, which was published in the *Archives of Internal Medicine*. Those living closer to fast-food restaurants ate more of it, especially low-income men. But the surprise was that easy access to supermarkets was not linked to a greater consumption of healthful foods.[32]

And easy access to supermarkets doesn't seem to help in the fight against obesity either. A larger study from NIH surveyed 13,000 children about their heights, weights and eating habits and looked for some correlation to types of food establishments. Neither fast food nor supermarkets nearby predicted weight patterns.[33]

Food deserts mean different things in different places. First, the vast majority of the studies on the relationship between food environment and obesity have been conducted in affluent settings, primarily North America, the UK, and Australia. What is called a food desert in the United States would likely look more like a food swamp to a person living in a Sudanese refugee camp.

For example, in Japan where obesity is only 3.4 percent, a lack of supermarket access doesn't predict obesity according to the Organisation for Economic Co-operation and Development health data. In fact, a food desert is more likely to be associated with undernutrition. Also, convenience stores and fast-food proximity don't seem to increase obesity in Japan. The country has plenty of McDonald's, but these outlets are less viewed as places for a fast snack or meal than a friendly place for hanging out and doing homework for school kids and a gathering place for older people.[34]

Food desert labels may be oversimplifying a big problem. Many things enter into a person's choosing healthy food: taste, price, and education, among others. In my neighborhood in Cairo, fresh grapefruits and oranges are squeezed into a glass for about 40 cents, while a stalk of sugar cane becomes a refreshing drink that costs less than half that. Which one do you think sells best in a poor country such as Egypt?

In any case, supermarkets, whether viewed as problem or problem-solver, are across the world now with huge growth in Latin America, Southeast Asia, China, and South Africa.[35] But what is more super than a supermarket? A big-box store, a wholesale club, or what the retail industry calls a supercenter.

Carrefour is such a place, a French supercenter rising out of the desert outside Cairo. During the 2011 revolution, vandals swept in and stole everything: laptops, televisions, housewares, clothes, and food. But Carrefour returned. It is busier than ever. A growing middle class throngs the aisles, filling fat cells and shopping carts with varieties of food never seen before. Of course, poor people come too, either by foot or a four-cent bus ride to stare and dream of pleasures of imported cheese and premium ice creams. Supercenters like Carrefour and its clones may be part of the obesity problem. Big boxes lead to big consumption. Supercenters have been accused of causing 10 percent of the rise in obesity since the 1980s. In a 2010 paper, two economists suggested that each "additional supercenter per 100,000 people increases . . . the obesity rate by 2.3 percentage points."[36]

Shoppers should be smarter than this. We can use plenty of tricks to fight the leviathan forces pressing us to buy and eat too much: Avoid shopping before lunch so that gummy bears and potato chips won't find their way into your cart. Bigger sizes sometimes make us eat more. You may only have to buy one to get that great deal on ten jars of mayonnaise. Hot dogs at Ikea smell better than they feel in the stomach.

But what about children? Young minds can't tell the difference between a Sesame Street nutrition jingle and a paid commercial for Frosted Flakes. Parents can turn off the television, of course, to resist the incessant junk food messages. They can avoid the candy aisle at the supermarket and steer away from the fattiest fast food. But what to do when the very institutions entrusted to educate their children and protect their health often fail?

Schools bargained with the junk food devil when they offered soda companies rights to their vending machines in return for money. Greg Critser, in his outstanding exposé on obesity called *Fat Land,* reveals how schools signed "pouring contracts":

> Such contracts typically involved three monetary perks for three contractual promises. For agreeing to sell, only, say, Coke, a school would receive commissions and a yearly bonus payment—sometimes as much as $100,000—to do with as it liked. In return for putting up Coke advertising around the campus, the school would receive free product to sell at fund-raising events. And in return for making the company's carbonated beverages available during all hours, Coke would provide additional "marketing" tools—banners, posters, etc.—to aid still more school fund-raising events. In a time of tight funds and rising expectations, such contracts proved enormously popular.[37]

Soda consumption soared. And even worse, it was replacing milk and other more healthful beverages.

At the same time, school lunch was changing dramatically. Pizza, tacos, and entire fast-food operations moved in. The lunch ladies, after all, were no longer volunteer moms; they ended up as cost centers, which would be downsized and replaced by processed convenience foods.

Not even the most enlightened schools get it. The nutrition committee in an international school in Berlin was warned not to act too fast. Candy, pastries, and sodas stayed at the lunch counter that year; the following year, the pastries moved behind the counter, but the other sweets remained out front.

And in Cairo, there is a kiosk outside my daughter's high school that sells soda, candy, chips, gum, cigarettes—the usual junk. Ten feet away are two teenaged military police armed with rifles, protecting the perimeter walls of the campus. Security is always a concern in Cairo these days, but school administrators should know this: junk food kills too; it just takes longer. These kiosks are the equivalent of 7-Elevens and other convenience stores in the United States. In fact, they may cause more obesity in teens than fast food according to new research from California. "A convenience store within a ten-minute walking distance of a school was associated with a higher rate of overweight students than schools without nearby convenience stores." In this survey, fast-food restaurants and supermarkets were not associated with obesity.[38]

Vending machines inside schools are part of the problem. Candy, chips, and sodas proliferate. In some schools, granola bars, pretzels, and energy drinks are substituted. The replacements are often as high in fats and sugars as the junk food booted out.

What about hospitals? Are hospitals the places to enforce good eating habits? Children's Hospital in Philadelphia had a McDonald's in its lobby. The Ronald McDonald House hosts families of sick children who need affordable places to stay near the hospital. It's hard to judge and even harder to criticize when very sick or terminally ill children grasped a bit of happy from the meals and colorful playground. But happy can also mean wholesome food.

And what are the rationalizations for what has become of the modern American drugstore? Behold the wonders: Potato chips, salted crackers, Pop-Tarts, sodas, premium ice creams, gumdrops, Twizzlers, chocolates, and seemingly any sweet produced from Switzerland to Amish country. All these greet the customer who stumbles through a game of reality Candyland.

Beyond this tempting gauntlet, the pharmacy desk is hidden at the back of these stores, ostensibly to discourage narcotic-seeking thieves. If the customer detours from the delectables aisles, she will find some over-the-counter solutions to those empty calories and unhealthy fats piled up in her cart. Terrific products, some of them, especially for people who choose to eat poorly: fiber pills and powders and all the various digestive aids for those suffering from constipation, diarrhea, reflux, and heartburn. And there are fat-dissolving aids, sugar-lowering pills, blood-pressure lowering minerals, cholesterol-lowering antioxidants—the list of remedies for the unhealthy lifestyle is long.

It is ironic that foods contributing to chronic diseases are marketed right next to the very products that may ease the problems. In some cases, both come from the same global food conglomerate. Yes, we've come a long way from the quaint apothecary serving up potions with a pestle. Too far, some may say: most other countries still keep pharmacies as separate entities. This practice of selling the cause and the cure side by side is unmistakable; look forward to liquor stores selling Viagra and cigarette machines offering bottles of cough syrup.

Snacking

Food is everywhere. Eating has become too convenient. In fact, we can do it anytime, which brings us to the next big change in the eating landscape of the past three decades that coincides with the rapid rise in obesity—snacking. Two forces led to this. First, time crunches as folks skipped breakfast, ate lunch at a desk, and grabbed something in front of a television or computer rather than sitting at the dinner table. And second, a vast array of high-calorie snacks invaded shelves. The sheer number and assortment led to higher intake, say obesity researchers. The urge to seek variety, once an evolutionary mandate, was now backfiring.

Wade Thoma for McDonald's said that items consumed between meal times have been the fastest-growing part of McDonald's business for three years, reported Julie Jargon of the *Wall Street Journal* in 2010. The most popular snack items were coffee drinks, smoothies, snack wraps, and desserts such as snack-sized McFlurry. The last supplies 340 calories, which is fewer calories and less than half the fat of the Angus Deluxe Snack Wrap.[39]

Over the last 30 years, the average number of snacks consumed per day has doubled, according to USDA data.[40]

Childhood trends are moving toward three snacks per day; over a quarter of children's daily calories come from snacks. Surveys of children in the United States show snacking surged from the late 1980s. While the biggest jump was in salty nibbles and candy intake, desserts and sugary beverages remain the major sources of calories from snacks. Childhood obesity rose in tandem with snacking. Some studies showed higher calorie intake and more obesity among snacking children, though some found a more even distribution of the energy intake throughout the day with lower body mass index. In any case, children are moving toward constant eating, a consumption pattern of three meals plus three snacks per day.[41]

Once considered a fresh diet concept—graze your way to your best weight—snacking is now considered one of the causes of the metabolic syndrome, a clutch of symptoms, including obesity, hypertension, and high blood sugar, which can lead to diabetes and heart disease.

Snacking is most popular among the poor. And no coincidence, they have more obesity and metabolic syndrome than higher income classes. A Taco Bell billboard urges us to stop in for a "fourth meal, the meal between dinner and breakfast." Or as UrbanDictionary. com defines it: "a corporate conspiracy to further addict the hapless masses to crappy, fat-laden food."[42] In late 2012, Taco Bell added churros and cookie sandwiches to its sweets menu of cinnamon twists and caramel apple empanadas. The plan is to market them as snacks rather than as desserts to follow meals.

Supersizing

As snacking grew, so did portion size.

A McDonald's employee urges you to supersize your order. As Critser reported in his book *Fat Land*, "A serving of McDonald's french fries had ballooned from 200 calories (1960) to 320 calories (late 1970s) to 450 calories (mid-1990s) to 540 calories (late 1990s) to the present 610 calories. In fact, everything on the menu had exploded in size." Critser explained that the recession of the mid-seventies set in motion a new concept to spur sales. Supersizing became the norm: A Double Gulp at 7-Eleven weighed in at 64 ounces but cost only a few pennies more than half the size. Burger King offered double cheeseburgers for a dollar, not much more than a solo. A full buffet at Chinese restaurants-with some offering over 250 dishes—can cost the same as a single order of moo shu pork. And this one tops them all: any size Slurpee for the same low price.[43] Talk about an offer you can't refuse. It worked. We bought the best deals, which were the biggest sizes. The supersizing marketing schemes sabotaged willpower by targeting our wallets. McDonald's knew labor was expensive whereas potatoes and soda syrup were cheap, costs that barely bounced when supersizing. Customers were spending only a little more but getting a lot more calories.

Did supersizing change how much people ate? You bet it did. Barbara Rolls and colleagues at Pennsylvania State University found that volunteers ate more as portion size increased, regardless of body mass index or whether they served themselves.[44]

Large portions proved to be an economic stimulus package for the food industry. Yet our bodies did not benefit. The supersized items were the unhealthiest kinds, the most processed, cheapest bastardizations of food: soda and fries. Thirty years ago, just as the obesity epidemic was ratcheting up, I did research on this topic, looking at the effect of nutrition advertising on fast food sales of french fries and soda. Little did I know then, when obesity rates were half of present day, that the problem would get much worse, and people would still be growing fat on these cheap junk foods, only now the portions are larger.

It isn't unfair to single out soda and fries. These two in particular have driven the obesity train all the way to the present epidemic.

Nearly half of all Americans drink at least one soda every day according to a Gallup poll in 2012.[45]

And what's wrong with that?

Empty calories, for one; a missed chance to boost health with vitamins, minerals, probiotics, or phytochemicals. And then there is the bad stuff. High phosphorus in soda replaces needed calcium and makes Swiss cheese of young bones. Calcium deficiency is linked to obesity. Sugar rots teeth. Caffeine makes kids, especially young boys, hyperactive. And as if that weren't enough, there is a more clandestine harm in soda, one that is mixed up in the obesity epidemic.

With lavish corn subsidies enacted in the last century, America was awash in corn. High-fructose corn syrup was invented. Beverage companies used high-fructose corn syrup to replace some sugar and regular corn syrup. It had two things the beverage companies preferred: it was cheaper and had a longer shelf life when added to pastries and processed foods. The table sugar and high-fructose corn syrup combo didn't hurt sales. Sweetener intake shot up significantly in the past four decades in the United States, mostly in soft drinks.[46]

Corn, rather than the fructose in syrup, may turn out to be the bigger problem concerning obesity. In addition to its invasion of the food supply from breakfast cereals to ketchup and most other processed foods, corn is also used as feed for pigs and cows like never before. The dangers of this will be covered in another chapter on food additives.[47]

Back to the most popular processed item: soda. Selling sugar water to the world has been a lesson in extraordinary marketing skill.

Coke has been in Africa since 1929 and is now in all of its countries; it is the continent's largest employer, with 65,000 employees and 160 plants, according to *BusinessWeek* magazine.[48] This is in spite of the fact that conducting business here is difficult because of war, poverty, and drought.

Kenya is one country that is trying its hardest to shed those burdens. Yet hunger is still a problem there, and obesity remains very low, at only 2 percent of the female population according to WHO 2010 databases. Make no mistake: Kenya is poor. Even people in the United States living below the poverty line are well off in comparison. Its capital city, Nairobi, hosts a vast slum called Kibera, where tin-roof shacks house as many as one million people. Raw sewage runs in the streets, and women line up to use a few latrines. Red Coca-Cola signs are everywhere. A bottle of Coke in these parts of Africa costs less than in New York City, but is still a big suck out of a daily wage, if a wage exists at all. According to Duane Stanford for *BusinessWeek*, "Coke is now in a street-by-street campaign to win drinkers, trying to increase per-capita annual consumption of its beverages in countries not yet used to guzzling Coke by the gallon. To do so, Coca-Cola is applying lessons learned in Latin America, where an aggressive courtship of small stores helped boost per-capita consumption in Mexico to the highest in the world." While Coke and Pepsi and other beverage companies point out that they have added calorie information and removed most of their products from schools, they continue a relentless push around the world.

How about fries with that Coke? French fries are similar in their fat profit margins. As we have seen, from the humble potato—boiled, mashed, or baked—has emerged a very lucrative spud when sliced and dipped in hot oil. Restaurants heaped the cheap commodity next to sandwiches and entrées; fast-food chains supersized them to the extent that a portion equaled nearly one-half of daily calorie requirements; big-box stores sold 10- and 20-pound bags at irresistible prices. The most consumed vegetable is a potato, largely due to its French connection. Each American eats more than 100 pounds of potatoes every year.[49]

Does it matter? If it weren't potatoes, it would be rice or noodles—so why blame the spud? Well, for one, fried rice and fried noodles share none of the modern ubiquity of french fries. And one damning piece of evidence against the potato comes from research that tracked over 120,000 people in Nurses' Health Study, Nurses' Health Study II, and the Health Professionals Follow-up Study, troves of health information gathered over many decades. The report examined lifestyle factors and weight gain every four years over 12 to 20 years. French fries topped the list for causing weight gain: an extra 3.4 pounds every four years. Potato chips notched second place, adding nearly 2 pounds to keep it all in the family. And to wash it all down, sugar-sweetened drinks ranked as the third most egregious food leading to extra pounds.[50]

French fries, chips, and soda: guilty as charged. Not all calories are created equal. Some are causing obesity.

ENTITLED TO JUNK FOOD

In Cairo, three out of four people eat subsidized foods. These commodities include flour, oil, sugar, and beans. Cheap sacks of sugar, gallons of clarified butter or palm oil called *ghee*, and daily bread called *aaysh* make certain the masses are fed. While the beans or *fuul* are healthful—except when drenched in oil—letting them eat cake is not. And apparently not a recipe for preventing revolutions.

The United States subsidizes farmers directly to produce corn and soy, two commodities that have crept into thousands of foods. They have to go somewhere. Yet Uncle Sam doesn't give incentives to the small farmer growing beans and tomatoes or the orchard owner harvesting apples. As a result, subsidies as they exist today may be adding to the world's obesity problem.

For poor Americans, another contributor may be the Supplemental Nutrition Assistance Program (SNAP), formerly known as the food stamp program. It is generous; the number of people receiving benefits has exploded: from 17 million people in 2000 to more than 47 million in 2013.[51] One of every 7 Americans receives free food every month, a benefit that allows them to use income on other essentials like rent and gas. A person receiving SNAP has a card similar to a debit card that has a monthly allowance for groceries. How much? In 2012, the average SNAP household received a monthly benefit of $272. A household of four could receive up to $668 monthly.[52]

According to the USDA, SNAP allows low-income people to buy the food they need for good health. Many go that route but many also buy soda, chips, and candy. SNAP participants consume less produce and healthy options and purchase at least 40 percent more sugar-sweetened beverages than any other consumer group.[53] While food restrictions are put on mothers getting benefits through Women, Infants, and Children (WIC), no such caveats come with SNAP.

Alarmed by obesity figures in New York City, Mayor Michael R. Bloomberg proposed barring food stamp users from buying soda and other sugary drinks with their benefits. In striking down the plan, Tom Vilsack, the secretary of agriculture, said, "We are confident that we can solve the problem of obesity." The mayor earlier had tried to impose a state tax on soda but failed.[54] And most recently, Mayor Bloomberg fought to limit sales of sweet beverages in many venues to no larger than 16 ounces. No go on that one either. The USDA doesn't allow prepared foods to be purchased with SNAP cards; however, an option allows states to permit restaurants to accept food stamps from people who are homeless, disabled, or elderly.[55]

As the economy worsens and the population ages and weakens, those numbers swell. Why shouldn't these individuals use their SNAP cards for a taco or fried fish sandwich? asks Yum! Brands, the parent company of Pizza Hut, Taco Bell, KFC, Long John Silver's, and A&W. The company has lobbied to have all food stamps be accepted at their restaurants. Dietitians strongly oppose the move.

Whether it is food stamps in the United States or subsidies in Egypt, such programs inadvertently increase obesity by missing a chance to boost healthy food intake. On one hand, the USDA promotes health with elaborate and costly nutrition programs and guidelines but then undermines it by allotting more than one-fifth of its budget to help produce foods it warns against, such as high-fructose corn syrup and hydrogenated oils.[56]

Do healthy foods cost more than junk foods? When apples at a big supermarket cost $2.99 a pound, and potato chips much less, it is a fair question. Mark Bittman reported in the *New York Times* that in recent decades, fresh produce prices have increased by 40 percent while the cost of soda and processed food has decreased by as much as 30 percent—all adjusted for inflation.

Yet Bittman argued: "The alternative to soda is water, and the alternative to junk food is not grass-fed beef and greens from a trendy farmers' market, but anything other than junk food: rice, grains, pasta, beans, fresh vegetables, canned vegetables, frozen vegetables, meat, fish, poultry, dairy products, bread, peanut butter, a thousand other things cooked at home—in almost every case a far superior alternative."[57]

At the risk of comparing apples and oranges, eating well for little is possible. The USDA spends millions publishing reports on how to put together a healthy menu on a budget. Eat fruits and vegetables in-season, cook in batches, buy loss-leaders . . . it absolutely can be done. But it takes a little time and a helping of patience, which fewer people seem to possess these days. Scrape the dirt off a carrot, slice it up—takes a minute more than ripping open a bag of baby carrots. It's not quite as easy or fast to eat healthy foods. But it can be cheaper than fast food and far tastier.

Still, soda and fries can taste pretty good. Why is that? The fact is, we are slaves to our evolutionary biology; sugar and fat are the go-to ingredients when we are hungry—they are the most nutrient dense. But what happened to our willpower? Why are we all such suckers for the stuff when we know they are making us fat and as intelligent mammals we know we don't need all those calories?

Sold on Junk Food

Simple: brilliant marketing. In addition to celebrity endorsements, emotional music, riveting commercials, and clever pricing models, aka Big Gulp, we are subjected to less-than-subtle product placement in movies, television, and at sporting events. And it's not fruits and vegetables being touted. An alarming 98 percent of food advertising to children in the United States is for items high in sugar, fat, and salt. In Europe, a few countries require advertisement-free television for kids, but most bombard viewers with ads for sugared cereals, soft drinks, candy, salty snacks, and fast-food outlets.[58]

The marketers are sly. They create confusion about nutrition when it is really very simple: "Eat food. Not too much. Mostly plants," as author and activist Michael Pollan nicely put it.[59] Marketers maintain, while cozying up to dietetic associations, that no food is bad and that every food fits on the nutrition pyramid or plate. The messages slide in with free gifts: Funds for schools that sell Pepsi in the cafeteria, money for college football teams that gulp Gatorade on the sidelines, and, in the most masterful stroke of all, toys for the youngest customers.

"Every month about 90 percent of American children between the ages of three and nine visit a McDonald's," wrote Eric Schlosser in his classic book *Fast Food Nation.*[60]

Most likely it is the toy, and not the Chicken McNuggets, they want. I know, because I bit for every Pokemon, Cabbage Patch, Tamogotchi, Disney character, and Furby—well, maybe not the homely Furby. But, bottom line, no one had to twist my arm—a dietitian's arm at that—because I liked the tie-ins: the toys were safe and durable for my children. According to Schlosser, a successful promotion doubles or triples the weekly sales volumes of children's meals. The legendary Teenie Beanie Baby promotion sent profits sky high: sales increased by nearly 1,000 percent, a phenomenally successful campaign. Word was that whole cartons of food were being trashed—by adult collectors. The valuable stuffed toys were yanked from Happy Meals like ivory tusks from elephants.

Acting like children? Hardly. Kids behave better. Young people eat food because it comes with a toy or sticker or colorful package. A study done at the Rudd Center for Food Policy and Obesity Research at Yale University tested that theory.

"Forty 4- to 6-year-old children tasted 3 pairs of identical foods (graham crackers, gummy fruit snacks, and carrots) presented in packages either with or without a popular cartoon character [like Scooby Doo, Dora the Explorer, and Shrek]. . . . Children significantly preferred the taste of foods that had popular cartoon characters on the packaging, compared with the same foods without characters."[61]

In an experiment done at Stanford University School of Medicine, children tasted foods and drinks in McDonald's packaging along with the identical ones in unbranded packaging. The preschoolers thought the branded ones tasted better.[62]

Money spent on food marketing is growing every year as are venues for ad placement; in addition to old-school ads including television commercials, movies, and billboards, subtle and not-so-subtle messages await in video games, smartphone apps, and the newest barrage from social media, whether through "likes" on Facebook or tweets from McDonald's.

The rise in food marketing mirrors the sharp increase in obesity in children. Since the 1970s, rates have more than doubled in preschoolers and tripled among six- to eleven-year-old children.[63]

The cool thing is that clever ads can work both ways. An Elmo sticker on a package of broccoli got more kids in one study to choose the vegetable over a chocolate bar. Without any stickers, over three-fourths chose the candy.[64]

And how about this ultimate marketing lure: playgrounds in fast-food places. Are they good or bad? Mothers in Cairo or Delhi—two crowded cities without much in the way of safe play places—find them a godsend. I was faithful fan for several years. As a mom with two toddlers in a place called Bucks County, a beautiful but isolated area above Philadelphia, I loved the indoor playground, especially on rainy days. McDonald's doesn't force you to buy french fries or make your kids drink soda from a sippy cup. In fact, they wouldn't boot you even if you came daily and bought nothing but a bottle of water. Oh, and the certain availability of bathrooms, especially in big cities and global sites, is a bonus for travelers and the bladder-challenged of all ages. That said, when your child sees every other kid diving into a Happy Meal, you may be buying a Happy Meal. In those days, carrot sticks were available in little pouches. Then they disappeared: not enough sales and too much spoilage. But in the twenty-first century, carrots are back, as well as raisins, apple slices, and orange segments depending on the time of year and the region in which they're being served. High-fiber oatmeal is showing promise.

McDonald's will respond to public sentiment, usually when expressed in an affidavit; they took the trans fats out of the fries as well as the scalding heat out of the coffee. By 2012, sizing was no longer super and mysterious pink slime (ammonia-treated beef) was shown the door.

This brings me back to my research decades ago measuring the effect of nutrition advertising on fast-food sales. I picked Arby's because they offered a mix of menu items and because there were two in my university town, I had a convenient control. A friend who was a talented artist designed wall boards depicting the virtues of milk versus soda and salad versus fries. The ads were big. The effect was small. Surveys showed that most went to Arby's for the fatty meal or snack; milk and salad were not going to entice them. Fast forward. Some campaigns have been successful in encouraging more healthful eating. One from Kellogg Company promoting high-fiber cereals saw an increase in sales.[65] Health claims on nutrition labels are one way to get the message out, but FDA and European Union regulations and fines have put a kink in some of those plans. Yogurt makers and others have had to rethink how to tell the public about health benefits of their products. Then certain unpackaged foods like fruits and vegetables get very little in the way of advertising dollars.

People may not want to pay extra for the good stuff. Though they tell researchers they would like to buy healthier foods, the reality may be different. Some of this is because the greasy stuff is cheaper and more heavily advertised, but it's also due to a fickle demand for healthy food. For example, the McDonald's near the Spanish Steps in Rome sported a salad bar replete with—I kid you not—a huge bowl of fresh strawberries. In Moscow and Tokyo and other prime global spots, fast-food restaurants bow to cultural differences.

Eating as Entertainment

Growing up, there were banana splits for good report cards, pizza parties to mark the beginning of vacation, and seafood splurges on New Year's Eve. Eating as celebration is as old as ham on Easter, lamb for Eid, and challah on Rosh Hashanah. These holidays—called occasions because they are infrequent events—haven't caused this epidemic of obesity. What we are seeing today is eating as entertainment, a dangerous hobby when there is so much leisure time to be filled. There are countless examples of this modern obsession with eating and food: Millions of websites and blogs devoted to the pleasures of food; young and old attending cooking schools in record numbers; celebrity cooks sending drooling fans to bookstores, where cookbooks outsell Pulitzer winners; chefs sculpting foam towers and spinning intricate nests from simple ingredients like kids with a can of Playdoh—with paintbrush and torch they can design a ten-inch dinner plate like a Caravaggio still life. What was once punishable—playing with your food—is now being lauded as art.

There is an ever-growing cult of restaurant-going, fueled by the reviews and discussion of Zagat, Yelp, and OpenTable. There are crazy theme restaurants: Dinner in the Sky in Belgium ("It's dining at altitude, and you're hoisted hundreds of feet in the air for a memorable experience where the view is unencumbered by annoying things like windows and a floor," writes Jason Arango for *dailyfork.com*); Modern Toilet in Taiwan ("food is served in plastic toilet bowls, to diners sitting atop toilet seats"); Sehnsucht in Germany (". . . geared toward anorexics. Menu items are given names that are in no way related to food so customers won't feel uncomfortable ordering"), and an even more disturbing concept, Khmer Rouge Experience Cafe in Cambodia, where diners presumably go hungry as did millions under the reign of terror there in the 1970s.[66]

While cooking shows on television are not new—consider Julia Child and Graham Kerr—the sheer number of them today reflects the pleasure we get in watching food in all its guises. Naked Chef, Iron Chef, Master Chef, and Great Chefs, as well as Rachel Ray, Two Fat Ladies, Emeril Lagasse, and Paula Deen are just a few of the on-air personalities. Food Network gives us 24-hour "food porn" as some in the media have described the habit of watching others cook on television or gazing at food dishes in glossy magazines. Food Network has as big an audience as CNN.

Food magazines are more popular than ever. Though *Gourmet*

magazine stopped publishing, hundreds more flourish. The gourmand philosophy grows shamelessly even as obesity rises. Television chefs build media empires with eponymous magazines, cookbooks, and kitchenware equipment for their fans. Many of these celebrity chefs, some overweight or obese themselves, encourage unhealthful eating by cooking with liberal amounts of butter, cream, and sugar, and, when not outwardly contemptuous of healthful eating, toss off a conspiratorial wink about its sinful pleasures. The audience is in on the joke, but it is no laughing matter when such habits add up to billions of pounds of excess fat. And in the case of Paula Deen, diabetes. Deen rolled out an endorsement of a Novo Nordisk diabetes management program to a vast crowd of dietitians at the Food and Nutrition Conference and Expo in 2012. Memory of her famous Lady's Brunch Burger—bacon and egg sandwiched between two glazed donuts—failed to dampen the applause.

It gets more ridiculous: A 130-pound man named Takeru Kobayashi dominated Nathan's Hot Dog Eating Contest until Joey Chestnut deposed him in 2007. Both can eat (which means not "chipmunking" or storing in the mouth) 59 of the sausages in 10 minutes. Joey won in overtime. The International Federation of Competitive Eating (IFOCE) hosts more than 100 such events every year. Whole beef tongue, bowls of mayonnaise, sticks of butter, and cow brains are among the foods inhaled at high-speed in absurd quantities. The IFOCE established eating as a sport in the 1990s and oversees competitive eating worldwide at the same time it licenses products and rallies its fan base with online videos. In 2002, Fox Network aired an eating contest called Glutton Bowl.[67]

The Japanese have a curious way with food. At one end we have massive sumo wrestlers fed like ducks fattened for fois gras. That's entertainment. And on the other we see the beautiful model of self-discipline called *hara hachi bu*, which means "Eat until you are only 80 percent full."[68] It is a practice that contributes to the extreme longevity of the Japanese people: Okinawa, Japan, has a higher percentage of centenarians than anywhere else in the world. Much of the endurance is attributed to their low rate of obesity, at less than 4 percent, and a diet high in fish and vegetables. *Hara hachi bu*. English has no such expression.

SOLUTIONS

Margaret Chan relates the following:

> Widespread obesity in a population is not a marker of failure of individual willpower, but of failure in policies at the highest level. Processed foods, very high in salt, trans fats, and sugar, have become the new staple food in nearly every corner of the world. They are readily available and heavily marketed. For a growing number of people, they are the cheapest way to fill a hungry stomach. The world certainly needs to feed its population of nearly 7 billion people. But it does not need to feed them junk food.[69]

The world has a big problem. Obesity is not going away; it is engulfing populations and public health budgets like few other diseases before it.

What to Do?

Advise people to stop eating so much? That route hasn't worked for many obese people; most regain the weight. Personal responsibility cannot be ignored or discounted but truth is, human biology hasn't changed much in the last three decades. What has changed is our environment. The solution lies with our surroundings, one that causes fat buildup at every turn. Obesity is the result of people responding normally to this fattening or obesogenic environment: one in which calorie-dense foods and beverages are tasty, cheap, and easy. While support for individuals such as nutrition education will be more vital in this climate, particularly in prevention, wide policy change is urgently needed to slim down our bloated cultures.

Where to begin? For starters, take a brief look at other public health campaigns that have been successful. In the early 1980s, hospitals in America were at the vanguard of persuading people to wear seat belts in cars and forgoing smoking in the office. The 450-bed teaching hospital where I worked dangled nice rewards (I won binoculars) for wearing a seat belt (they put checkpoints in the hospital parking lot). The hospital administration gave people one month to quit smoking inside the building and relegated holdouts either to the loading dock or a small smoky chamber in shameful view of the rest of the employees. The campaign was a phenomenal success in changing behaviors. And it was accomplished using principles of Child Psychology 101: firm rules tempered with reward and punishment.

All across the land, similar programs and new laws were prompting citizens to stomp out cigarettes and strap on seat belts. Joe Camel was no longer welcome. Threat of dismissal, cold shoulders, advertising restrictions, and fines swiftly turned the tide on two big public health issues: today nearly 85 percent of Americans wear seat belts regularly, and smoking has been cut in half.

Obesity will be a bigger challenge.

Because we must eat to survive, we can't go cold turkey. Shifting food behaviors is far more complex. And when it comes to food, good and bad are not black and white.

Many countries are taking steps, while others are just waking to the deluge of chronic health problems headed their way. Brazil has been exemplary: it introduced national monitoring programs, restrictions on marketing to children, and improved school food. In the United States, the White House Task Force on Childhood Obesity is developing a national action plan, while Michelle Obama has spearheaded a campaign to encourage healthier food in schools, better food labeling, and more physical activity for children. In Egypt, where obesity in women matches the 48 percent rate in the United States, health officials are overwhelmed by this new epidemic because they also continue to struggle with millions of stunted and undernourished children.

Policy change reaches more people and lasts longer. Obesity experts agree that laws and regulations must evolve. However, they are also difficult to pass and are at the mercy of partisan politics and powerful food lobbies.[70]

For instance, who is to say that a milkshake from Wendy's should be singled out for tax instead of a smoothie from McDonald's? A Triscuit versus a Saltine? A Red Bull versus a Coke Zero? Regulators everywhere are feeling the collective migraine.

Nevertheless, here are a few ideas gaining traction in the anti-obesity fight.

Taxes on Unhealthy Foods

Public health experts are pushing for a tax on sugary soft drinks. A penny an ounce, which is being proposed, would raise billions of dollars for health care. Obesity researcher Kelly Brownell, as director of the Rudd Center for Food Policy and Obesity at Yale, has advocated for such a levy since the 1990s. The powerful beverage lobby had easily fought such a tax, invoking discrimination and personal rights. Wrote Brownell with city of New York health commissioner Thomas R. Frieden in 2009:

> Objections have certainly been raised: that such a tax would be regressive, that food taxes are not comparable to tobacco or alcohol taxes because people must eat to survive, that it is unfair to single out one type of food for taxation, and that the tax will not solve the obesity problem. But the poor are disproportionately affected by diet-related diseases and would derive the greatest benefit from reduced consumption; sugared beverages are not necessary for survival; Americans consume about 250 to 300 more calories daily today than they did several decades ago, and nearly half this increase is accounted for by consumption of sugared beverages; and though no single intervention will solve the obesity problem, that is hardly a reason to take no action.[71]

As obesity and its enormous cost in health care mounts, the discussion is resonating. Brownell says the tax would reduce soft drink consumption as well as help fund Medicare and Medicaid. But what would be a win-win for health would be a fall in profits for beverage companies. Americans Against Food Taxes, a new organization heading the response and paid for by the beverage industry, is buying full-page newspaper ads and television time. Policy makers concede that it will be a tough battle, but they suggest that states and cities should begin, much the way tobacco taxes spread.

Removing sugary drinks in schools, as some districts have done, hasn't cut down total sugar consumption from beverages, as expected. Teenagers still drink about 15 percent of their daily calories. The study published in the *Archives of Pediatrics and Adolescent Medicine* looked at thousands of public school students across 40 states. It found that removing soda from cafeterias and school vending machines only prompted students to buy sports drinks, sweetened fruit drinks, and other sugar-laden beverages instead.[72] This recent finding adds urgency to a call for other ways to curb unhealthy eating such as more comprehensive bans as well as taxes.

In 2013, Suzanne Daley of the *New York Times* wrote about food taxes in Europe:

> France, Finland, Denmark, Britain, Ireland and Romania have all either instituted food taxes or have been talking about it. But perhaps no country is trying harder than Hungary, which has, in the past 18 months, imposed taxes on salt, sugar and the ingredients in energy drinks, hoping both to raise revenues and force those who are eating unhealthy foods to pay a little more toward the country's underfinanced health system.

Officials told Daley that sales of salty and sugary foods have dropped in the last year. "But it is hard to tell if the taxes had much to do with it. Hungarians, struggling with high unemployment and a dismal economy, bought less of all kinds of foods last year," she wrote.[73]

Subsidies for Healthy Foods

Subsidies work the opposite of taxes. They encourage consumption because they artificially deflate prices. Egypt is a good example. The government ensures that the staples including bread, sugar, oils, and lentils are affordable for all. Bread costs *piasters*, or pennies, a good thing in a land where 40 percent make less than the equivalent of two dollars a day. People complain about the price of chicken and say lamb and beef are out of reach, so they fill themselves with fat and carbohydrate calories. Yet, as said before, a vast majority of Egyptian women are overweight or obese. Using data on price and consumption changes, one researcher asked if Egyptian taxes and subsidies were partly to blame. The findings indicated that government subsidies for bread and sugar may have contributed to an obesity epidemic in Egypt.[74]

The United States has made similar missteps. The Farm Bill, which is rewritten every five years or so, gives billions of dollars to farmers to grow soybeans and corn. No such incentives are given for fruits or vegetables. As a result, industry has been flooded with cheap commodities—high-fructose corn syrup, for example—which have worked their way into soft drinks, breads, crackers, and countless processed foods. Included in these massive bills are the funds and rules for the Supplemental Nutrition Assistance Program (SNAP), formerly known as Food Stamps. When one in seven Americans is receiving government money for food each month, and obesity keeps rising, it is time to assess what foods are being bought, say experts. The SNAP program currently provides low-income households with electronic debit cards to use for the purchase of eat-at-home foods. Hence, one policy idea is that when the card is used to buy a healthy food, the cardholder should be charged only a share of the cost, whereas when unhealthy food is bought, the cardholder could be charged extra. A pilot study in Massachusetts is offering SNAP recipients a 30 percent subsidy on produce for 15 months.[75]

Will changing the price of unhealthy foods change weight? Taxes and subsidies can work. In 2008 the WHO recommended that policy should encourage healthy eating.

Economists and obesity researchers have wrestled with price elasticity models. Anne Marie Thow and colleagues reviewed how changing prices may affect diet and obesity for the Bulletin of the World Health Organization.[76]

These are a few predictions they uncovered:

- 27% tax on soda prices in Norway = 44% decrease in heavy users.

- 20% tax on salty snack foods in the US would reduce energy intake only about 830 calories per person per year.

- 10% tax on cheese and butter and other high-fat products in France = weight loss of 1.3 kilograms (2.87 lbs.) per year.

Researchers at the Institute for Health Research and Policy and Department of Economics at the University of Illinois predicted that small taxes or subsidies are not likely to produce significant changes in obesity prevalence but larger levies may, especially with young and low-income people.[77]

In a later review, 11 of 14 models estimated health benefits for lower-income groups. One objection to such taxes is that they penalize lower-income groups, but the health benefits should offset this.[78]

Other health researchers are against a "sin tax" for unhealthy foods because it may push people to choose other equally caloric but untaxed beverages such as smoothies, thereby not resulting in change to obesity rates.[79]

Denmark repealed a tax on high fat foods after just one year. Though the tax raised millions in revenue, the health effect was muted when citizens shopped across the border.[80]

What then if we made some healthy food free? Another program Fresh Fruit and Vegetable Program in the United States—healthy foods for low-income schoolchildren—reached annual funding of $150 million in 2011. It may pay for itself in reduced health care costs.

Making fresh fruits and vegetables more available is the concept behind Green Cart, a New York City initiative that puts healthy food within reach of more people by licensing up to 1,000 street vendors.[81] Then there are the small corner stores that compete with both carts and chain convenience stores. The Healthy Corner Store Initiative begun in Philadelphia is using grants and committed workers to motivate small stores to put more nutritious foods on shelves.[82]

Role for Food Industry

In 2002, two obese teenagers in the Bronx borough of New York City sued McDonald's for deceptive marketing. The suit claimed that McDonald's failed to disclose the ingredients in their fare, much of which is high in fat, salt, sugar, and cholesterol. The plaintiffs argued that McDonald's should therefore be held accountable for the girls' obesity, heart disease, diabetes, high blood pressure, and high cholesterol.

The case was thrown out of court.

Litigation exposes wrongdoing. But it is difficult to blame one food for obesity since people eat a variety of food. The exception would be Morgan Spurlock, who ate his way through a month of supersized McDonald's meals and had high cholesterol, weight gain, and the award-winning documentary *Super-Size Me* to show for it.[83] Lawsuits may not be a solution here, as they were in tobacco industry, where million dollar settlements forced industry changes.

The food industry will respond voluntarily to show good faith and prevent strict regulation. A good example is the 2011 Kids Live Well Initiative, an agreement among 19 fast food chains including Burger King, IHOP, and Chili's (with the glaring exception of McDonald's) to have more healthful menu options for children.[84]

Another example has to do with trans fats—the harmful synthetic fat used to make margarine and crisp crackers, which last longer on store shelves. Though many companies dragged their feet, the troublesome fats have finally been removed from most products. While the government of New York City ordered its removal, many companies did so voluntarily.

Healthy foods are better for our bottoms, to be sure, and now food companies are finding that they also add to their bottom lines. Analysts report that healthy products including yogurts and whole grains are churning a higher share of profits. The report looked at products and earnings at 15 major food companies, including Kraft, Heinz, General Mills, and Coca-Cola.[85]

That should make their marketing job a bit easier. One of the reasons the Bronx case was thought frivolous or nuisance was because McDonald's offers nutrient information for all their menu items. The plaintiffs should have known that a ten-piece Chicken McNuggets had 470 calories and 30 grams of fat.

Food companies in many countries are required to put nutrition labels on products. Cities and states are now demanding that restaurants label menu items.

Chefs and owners are scared to death. Restaurants across the spectrum of Michelin star ratings can no longer hide: from the liberal use of butter and salt at the high-end to the deep-fried padding common in chain restaurants, damage done by eating out will be exposed.

New York City requires restaurants to post calorie labels. Will it make a difference? A 2011 study published in the *International Journal of Obesity* examined the impact of calorie labels on young people's fast-food choices in low-income communities in New York

City and in Newark, New Jersey.[86] Study restaurants included four of the largest chains in those cities: McDonald's, Burger King, Wendy's, and Kentucky Fried Chicken.

Results? Though over half noticed the new labels, there was no difference in choice because of them.

Other states report better response to labels. Results from a recent study conducted in New Haven, Connecticut, found that restaurant diners consumed fewer calories when item calorie labels were included on the dinner menu and 14 percent fewer calories when the recommended daily calorie intake for the average adult was also printed on the menu.[87]

Making nutrition information available and user-friendly may work best for consumers who are already nutrition conscious.[88] When people can plainly see the calorie and fat content on their plates or in their takeout bag, they should "vote with their fork," as nutrition expert Marion Nestle advised.

Some advocates think industry is more culpable. One proposal would be to assign a target for each fast-food or sugary beverage business, much like a person or corporation keeps defined sections of highways clean and landscaped in the United States. Each company would be responsible for lowering childhood obesity in a specific area. For example, McDonald's based in Chicago would be assigned the midwestern states, whereas Coca-Cola's turf would be the southeastern region, which includes their home offices in Atlanta. The government would penalize them if they did not reach goals.[89]

One ambitious project introduced by Healthy Weight Commitment Foundation (HWCF) has major food and beverage companies pledging to cut a combined 1.5 trillion calories from their products by 2015. HWCF members, including Kellogg, Hershey, and Coca-Cola, accounted for a quarter of all calories consumed in the United States in 2007. The pledged reduction will whittle 0.8 percent of calories sold across the packaged food and beverage marketplace as well as reveal how changes in the food supply will effect individual diets, according to a paper coauthored by global nutrition expert and the plan's chief evaluator, Barry Popkin, at the University of North Carolina.[90]

These ideas ask that the food industry take responsibility for consequences of the products from which they profit.

Limit Advertising

Junk food advertising dwarfs that spent on fruits and vegetables. Bans on advertising to children—who cannot differentiate paid ads from facts—have helped. Governments can go further. Of course angering the food industry is not the goal of government because lobbies and PAC monies are what keep people in their elected jobs. Nevertheless, the Center for Science in the Public Interest in Washington, DC, is pushing for change. This nutrition watchdog has recently focused on obesity in countries like South Africa, joining with international activists for a Global Dump Soft Drinks Campaign.[91] The Walt Disney Company has taken a brave step toward eliminating advertising of less-than-nutritious foods to children. With a target date of 2015, all products pitched on their television shows, radio programs, and websites will pass a nutrition test. Michelle Obama hailed the initiative: "Disney is doing what no major media company has ever done before in the US—and what I hope every company will do going forward."[92]

Reduce Access

Schools have pulled sodas and chips from vending machines and woven healthier foods into cafeteria breakfasts and lunches. It may be working. A recent report from California said that students there were consuming fewer calories than in states without the changes.[93]

"The Healthy Food Financing Initiative supports projects that increase access to healthy, affordable food in communities that currently lack these options." Several United States agencies will "[develop] and [equip] grocery stores, small retailers, corner stores, and farmers markets selling healthy food."[94]

Burger King took another promising action: default items in kid's meals aren't soda and fries, which instead must be requested. Eighteen other restaurant chains joined the Kids Live Well campaign "to offer at least one children's meal that has fewer than 600 calories, no soft drinks, and at least two healthy food items," reported Sharon Bernstein for the *Los Angeles Times*.[95] And then of course, bold laws from Mayor Bloomberg in New York City hope to put enormous sugary drinks out of reach.[96]

Nothing Succeeds like Success

Thin people. How do they avoid the barrage of junk food choices? Why is Colorado the thinnest state in the United States and Mississippi the heaviest? How do Asians prevent weight gain when they move to Western countries like the United Kingdom? In a question: how do thin people confront a toxic food culture?

Following the lead of the positive psychology movement, which studies happiness, obesity researchers are asking thin people how they stay that way.

People who manage their weight well adopt lifelong habits—not a short stint on a diet—including exercising, keeping a food diary, and jumping on a scale once or twice a week. And germane to the toxic environment, they do the following: steer clear of buffets and all-you-can-eat situations, remove tempting foods like chips and ice cream from their kitchens, and avoid dining out too frequently and plan ahead when they do. Thin people—all but the most fidgety—work at keeping off the pounds the environment induces. It takes extreme vigilance in our modern world to prevent weight gain.

Humans are hard-wired to choose instant gratification (tasty, cheap, and easy) over long-term benefit, and they are also sponges for the marketing that creates desire in the first place. People do not choose to be obese.

The food industry deflects blame by framing the obesity problem as one of personal choice and parental failure. Officials like Mayor Bloomberg who propose soda taxes or food stamp restriction are lambasted as architects of a nanny state. Meanwhile, obesity is getting worse. Education has its important place, but stronger measures are needed as well. Obesity experts and activists say it is time to address the toxic environment. Whether through taxes, subsidies, or a good old-fashioned Twitter campaign, there is no time to waste.

7

· · · ·

FAT IS CONTAGIOUS: MICROBES & OBESITY

A fat-inducing virus may be making obesity as widespread as the common cold.

THE DRAGONFLIES SCOOPED FROM TWO PONDS near Pennsylvania State University met their fate only hours later. Decapitated, gutted, and dissected, these guys—all male *Libellula pulchella* types—gave their bodies to science in the unlikeliest of quests: the war against obesity.

Incredible as it sounds, dragonflies can get fat. But it is not from the many mites and mosquitoes on which they snack. Rather, a common intestinal parasite called *gregarine* is thought to be the culprit. Dragonflies infected with gregarine behaved much like slackers of the human species: they lazed around, lost wing strength, and shunned territorial flight contests with other males. As a result, their luck with the ladies took a dive. The problem? The dragonflies' wings had grown heavy with fat; like failed deicers, their muscles could no longer oxidize fatty acids. And without fatty acids for fuel, these Romeos lost lift midflight.

Researchers also observed that the listless dragonflies showed resistance to insulin, mirroring humans having metabolic syndrome.

Quick review: Central obesity plus any two of these four risk factors constitute a diagnosis of metabolic syndrome: raised triglycerides, reduced high-density lipoprotein cholesterol, raised blood pressure, or raised fasting blood sugar. Blood sugar (mostly trehalose in insects) was double that of healthy dragonflies. And when injected with insulin, the infected insects showed none of the expected drop in blood sugar.[1]

More disconcerting than diabetic dragonflies, however, is what this means for us: infections can cause obesity. It is a depressing development for sure. Personal experience had suggested that one could count on a stuffy nose or a touch of stomach flu to rein in appetite and drop a few pounds in the process.

Not true. Gut disturbances trigger fat deposits and other metabolic changes, according to the Penn State researchers. Whether the blame should go to the gregarine bugs themselves or the microbial mess they leave behind isn't certain.

This chapter takes a look at one more reason that obesity is epidemic: it's contagious. Though the John Galts of this world will argue that this is rationalization for poor self-control, the proof is mounting on two fronts. Microbiologists are churning out smart evidence-based research in the lab at the same time behavioral scientists are finding that obesity can be every bit as contagious as a yawn.

First, take a look at the discoveries that will have you shaking your head instead of hands.

CAN A BUG CAUSE OBESITY?

Say you catch a cold. Several days of sniffles and sneezes and soon you're good as new. Think again. A few cold viruses can leave behind lasting damage in a cellular hit-and-run, which in this case amounts to a pileup of fat cells. Dents in the smooth operation of fat metabolism remain long after the virus has fled the scene.

One cold virus in particular, adenovirus 36 (Ad-36), has been scrutinized in both animals and humans. Chickens, mice, and monkeys all show jumps in body fat when given this virus, even though they ate no more than the animals not exposed.[2]

It's tougher to study the effect in humans for several reasons. Infecting humans for research purposes is unethical, as was conceded much too late in Guatemala where in the 1940s, hundreds of prisoners were injected with syphilis for a United States study on penicillin.[3] And even if volunteers were forthcoming, obesity can be insidious, taking a period of time to develop. Fortunately, a simple method can be used to see who has been exposed: a blood test. Humans who have been exposed will have antibodies to the virus (the normal immune system response). A study conducted by Richard Atkinson and colleagues across three cities in the United States tested more than 500 obese and normal weight volunteers for antibodies to the Ad-36 virus. Just 11 percent of non-obese harbored the antibodies, but 30 percent of the obese did.[4]

A look for Ad-36 in children came up with a similar ratio. Exposure to the virus was seen in 22 percent of obese children but only 7 percent of normal-weight children.[5]

While many researchers agree on the solid connection between viruses and obesity, some are wary, citing the classic "chicken or egg" riddle. Instead of the virus causing obesity, could it be the reverse? Could obesity, by weakening the immune system, make the obese more vulnerable to the Ad-36 virus? One novel study addressed this question and found that two viruses not associated with obesity, Ad-2 and Ad-31, showed up equally in obese and normal-weight groups. Obese people were no more likely to contract these viruses than lean people, which suggests that Ad-36 may be the cause and not the result of obesity.[6]

When twins can be used in studies, it adds a bonus control because they share many genes. Another study by Atkinson and colleagues looked at Ad-36 in twins. The twins with the Ad-36 virus were heavier and fatter compared to their virus-free counterparts.[7]

And a 2012 meta-analysis from the University of Tokyo in Japan looked at ten studies from around the world and confirmed that Ad-36 was associated with risk of obesity and weight in humans.[8]

If Ad-36 does in fact make people fatter, how does it do it? Good question with a crazy complicated answer better suited to a textbook. But here goes, verbatim from "Ten Putative Contributors to the Obesity Epidemic," the seminal 2009 collaboration from 22 researchers around the world, from Kentucky to New Zealand:

> This virus enhances differentiation and lipid accumulation of 3T3-L1 and human primary preadipocytes . . . Ad-36 activates phosphotidyl inositol kinase (PI3K) and cAMP pathways,

increases cell replication, expression of several genes of adipogenic cascade such as PPARγ, CEBP/β and consequentially, induces differentiation and lipid accumulation in 3T3-L1 cells and human adipose derived stem cells (hASC). . . . Moreover, Ad-36 reduces leptin expression and secretion in rodent fat cells, which may reduce the autocrine/paracrine inhibitory effect of leptin on preadipocyte differentiation. . . . In-vitro infection with Ad-36 increases glucose uptake by primary rodent adipocytes and human adipose tissue explants or hASC human primary skeletal muscle cells through a virally induced increase in PI3K activation [9]

Got that? Here's the rough translation: Adenovirus 36, a common cold virus, can:

- Increase size and number of fat cells
- Reduce hormones including leptin
- Fuel enzymes to make more fat cells
- Transfer more sugar into fat cells

So here is a virus that—unlike chocolate cake, which leads to chubby but tastes good in the process—sabotages our figures in addition to stuffing up our sinuses. With such poor manners, this virus would be missed by no one. A vaccine eradicating this contagion would be welcome, but that solution has one problem.

Ad-36 isn't the only virus linked to obesity in humans. Two other viruses are known: Ad-37 and Ad-5.

In animals, as many as five viruses are involved. These have sprawling names to match their effects: canine distemper virus, Rous-associated virus type 7, Borna disease virus, scrapie agent, and SMAM-1.

The first four attack the central nervous system, while SMAM-1 is a virus from India that turns directly into fat cells.[10]

Here are the first four viruses and their modus operandi, condensed from the previously mentioned review by McAllister and colleagues.

- *Canine distemper virus* (CDV) fattens mice after the acute phase of the infection is done. CDV appears to promote weight gain by acting on hormones and leptin receptors.

- *Rous-associated virus-7* (RAV-7) causes obesity in chickens, possibly by decreasing thyroid hormones.

- *Borna disease virus* goes to work by damaging the hypothalamus and neuroendocrine systems in rats.

- *Scrapie agents* cause obesity in mice by derailing glucose in the brain.

- And the fifth, *SMAM-1*, acts directly on fat cells.[11]

From his early observations on chickens in India, graduate student Nikhil Dhurandhar followed the thread from Bombay in the late eighties to Pennington Biomedical Research Center in Louisiana, where he has coined the term "infectobesity."[12]

While infectobesity sounds like a spooky slogan for a new age, the underlying science is rigorous enough to appear across a spectrum of respected medical journals.

"Clinicians should be aware of infectobesity (obesity of infectious origin), and its potential importance in effective obesity management," concluded Dhurandhar in *Lancet Infectious Diseases* in 2011.[13]

As we saw in dragonflies, viruses and other agents can damage metabolic systems. But it is important to remember the exceptions: Not everyone with antibodies as a sign of exposure to these pathogens gained weight. And reversing it, not all overweight people have been exposed to the virus.

Dhurandhar also claims, "Clearly, not every case of obesity is of infectious origin. However, if a few pathogens can cause obesity, there may be more awaiting discovery. These data give a new perspective to the etiology of obesity and raise the possibility of infection as a contributing factor for obesity in some humans. When such a relationship between pathogens and human obesity is well established, vaccines or antimicrobial agents may be employed to prevent or treat some forms of obesity."[14]

Certain microbes can cause adipose tissue expansion, perhaps to contain infection, asserts Dhurandhar in a paper he published with colleague Vijay Hegde in 2013. The opposite is also true: obesity can increase our susceptibility to infection. Immunity suffers in the obese. Turns out adipose tissue is packed with more than just excess energy. Inside this dynamic mass are several types of cells including immune cells and stem cells, which may become either fat cells or immune cells. Obesity may convert the undecided stem cells into fat at the expense of immune cells. Also natural killer T cells, which kill pathogens, are reduced in obesity. Suboptimal immune response in the growing numbers of obese in the global population may have consequences in the event of influenza or other infectious disease epidemics.[15]

MICROBES

Viruses aren't the only unseen diet saboteurs. Consider their cousins: the 1,000-plus different species of microbes in the gut, some of which do an estimable job of squeezing out every last carbohydrate and fat gram from your lunch. Their miserly talents to extract energy or hamper expenditures as the CPAs of microbes may determine whether you, the host, is fat.

Who invited them? You did, at birth. Your Apgar wailing announced fresh meat, and the microbes descended, anxious to colonize a new world. That was with a cesarean section. If delivered naturally, your mother's birth canal was the first place microbes jumped aboard. And this is where it gets even more intriguing: if delivered by cesarean, newborns miss out on the mother's mix of microbes and instead populate with pirate microbes: those belonging to the obstetrician, a nurse, or the fellow mopping the floor. Which is not to say that these workers don't possess perfectly fine sets of microbes, but wouldn't it make more sense for your baby to have your bacteria, considering that your baby will be going home into your environment? Science and nature conspire in the birth canal, even as the fetus slips from womb to the world, to protect life.

Early microbiota impact later well-being. A healthy mix of microbes in infancy depends on the mode of delivery and quality of breast milk. When the blend is a mess, problems arise, especially in the inflammatory sphere. Obesity is one such problem.[16]

Erika Isolauri of the University of Turku in Finland said at a conference in Australia: "The good bacteria that babies pick up during the natural birth process play an important role in reducing an infant's risk of becoming overweight or obese in their early years of life."[17]

Unfortunately, cesarean sections are wildly popular. Rates have nearly doubled in the last decade, most markedly in high-income countries. (In poor countries, more sections could be done to prevent harm for mother and child.) One in three mothers in the United States now gives birth this way.[18] Brazil, Italy and Mexico are among the countries that do even more.[19] This trend may be a contributor to obesity, say researchers. A 2012 Harvard study found this to be the case. Cesarean section was chosen by 284 of 1255 Boston area women. By age three, 15.7 percent of the children delivered this way were obese compared with 7.5 percent of children born vaginally. Cesarean delivery doubled the odds of obesity.[20]

Infants delivered this way have fewer bifidobacteria and bacteroides, which seem to protect against obesity.

In addition to mode of delivery, another choice shapes the gut microflora during infancy: breast or bottle.

Breast milk delivers an exquisite mix of prebiotics, probiotics, and some yet unidentified compounds. While formula delivered in a bottle may be the next best thing, breast will always be best (except of course if a chance of transmitting a serious disease or drug dependence is present). Breast milk matches the baby's needs. It contains lactic acid bacteria and high numbers of bifidobacteria, which seem to be the ideal for baby.

Bifidobacteria may make the difference. Normal weight children at ten years of age had more bifidobacteria in their guts when they were three months old, compared to obese children, according to research from the University of Turku in Finland.[21]

Breast milk better protects against early infections, both gastrointestinal and respiratory. Breast milk changes the immune system. And as noted before, immune response is intimately related to adipose tissue.

Obesity results from too much energy coming in and not enough going out. While eating too much and moving too little obviously fits here, many other scenarios chip away at the equation. Even mindful eaters and stalwart exercisers report difficulty in maintaining calorie balance. Their guts tell them something is wrong and as it turns out, guts may be a source of the obesity problem, as well as a solution.

Growing evidence suggests that among the factors contributing to the host response toward nutrients, the gut microbiota represent an important one. We have more than 10^{14} bacteria in our gut; this translates into 100-fold more genes than our entire human genome.[22] These legions of squatters—or their numbers may suggest that we are alive at the mercy of these Lilliputians—aren't sitting around figuring out how to make us happy. These wee ones are clinging for dear life to the slippery pink membranes of our intestines. By and large it is a fair exchange. We supply the climbing wall and some snacks—indigestible leftover fibers for which we have no other use. As we shall see, we have the power to wash the whole harmonious community out at any time through changes in diet, medications, and more. Unfortunately, there can be payback. Some organisms such as *Clostridium difficile* can embed while wearing spores like Kevlar vests; few antibiotics can touch them. The resulting diarrhea and weight loss kills many thousands of people every year.[23] Some bacteria are double agents, friendly one day and upsetting stomachs the next. Others are quite greedy, grabbing and storing calories for us.[24] What may have been a lifesaving benefit hundreds of years ago is now making us obese.

To be sure, microbes should not be ignored. Our microbes can make us fat. This exciting area of research offers the following:

- Gut microbes can squeeze more calories from food.[25]
- Gut microbes can push storage of those calories as fat.[26]
- Lean and obese humans differ in numbers of two major bacteria, *Bacteroides* and *Firmicutes*.[27]
- Gut microbes are linked to both inflammation and the metabolic syndrome, prominent players in the obesity game. Increased intestinal permeability is one reason.[28]

Let's start with mice, from which prodigious discovery springs.

Germ-free mice have taught us much, particularly in the fields of genetics, immunology, and nutrition. Germ-free or gnotobiotic mice are special; it is not easy "creating" these animals. After the moms deliver by cesarean or "cervical dislocation," during which the moms are sacrificed, the pups are raised in sterile housing and fed sterile food and water throughout their short lives. Being germ-free, these bubble boys of the animal kingdom would appear to be shielded from all of life's slings and arrows of dirty infiltrators like flu bugs and the common cold.

But these animals are not healthy. They are fragile and highly susceptible to infection and disease once exposed. Microbes are vital for normal gastrointestinal and immune function as well as normal digestion of nutrients. But scientists did notice one perk of growing up germless. A big one.

If these germ-free mice were to escape and hightail it to the nearest fast-food dumpster, they would be well-equipped to face the modern diet with all its excesses. It seems the chow equivalent of greasy hamburgers and fries doesn't make these pups fat. Billion-dollar patent alert: Germ-free mice are resistant to obesity. In contrast to normal mice with a normal gut microbiota, germ-free animals are protected against obesity that develops after consuming the equivalent of a Western-style, high-fat, sugar-rich diet.

In a groundbreaking series of experiments, researchers at Washington University School of Medicine at St. Louis in Missouri fed normal and germ-free mice the same food for the first few months of their lives. The mice with microbes gained weight at a much faster clip even though they ate less food than their germ-free counterparts. And they had a 42 percent higher body fat. Gene for gene, these mice were carbon copies, except for one difference: their gut microbes. The researchers realized microbes were involved.[29]

Then they tried something else. They put the regular stew of microbes from the normal mice into the lean germ-free mice. Can you guess what happened? After just two weeks, body fat soared by 60 percent, and they weren't eating more. They were actually eating less. And exercise habits hadn't changed.

Not only did the mice get pudgy, they also developed insulin resistance, bigger fat cells, and changes in hormones including leptin.

In a separate study designed to find out what was causing this resistance to obesity in germ-free mice, the researchers found that the germ-free animals were spared because of two independent mechanisms.[30] Gut microbiota change both sides of the energy balance equation: first by influencing energy harvest from the diet, and second by affecting genes that regulate how energy is expended and stored.

More recently, researchers at the same university planted human microbes (via fresh or frozen stool) into these germ-free mice. Then they experimented with different diets: first, one high in fibrous polysaccharides, similar to what vegans or horses may eat, and afterward a swap to one high in fat and sugar, a typical modern diet. The researchers knew the mice would become obese, but they wanted to see what impact the diet switch had on their microbes. What they found was that the microbe community responded astonishingly fast to a change in diet—within one day.[31]

Our microbes outnumber us ten to one. Even with those odds, the microscopic Davids cooperate with Goliath; our small partners coevolved to forge mutually beneficial relationships. We share food. In repayment for our fruitful foraging (shopping at the supermarket), our microbial mates eat our table scraps and stockpile leftovers in our fat cells. This ability to store energy would be valuable in the old days when food wasn't just steps away, but in modern times, this benefit is decidedly unfriendly.

We know why they do it: A dead host is not making canapés. It is in microbes' best interest to keep us alive and full of fat. But how do they accomplish this? If we can figure out how it is done, maybe we can figure out how to undo it.

Microbes work several angles of the energy equation. This is what science has come up with:

Gut microbes harvest more from our food. Microbes eat stuff we can't digest. Microbes ferment indigestible polysaccharides to absorbable forms. And they sponge up more simple carbohydrates and short-chain fatty acids. In other words, they can eke out more calories ounce for ounce. A soda may mean 150 calories for me but 160 calories for someone else. The difference may be determined by our unique set of microbes.

How do we know this? Special mice have been genetically altered to be obese. They are called ob/ob mice. Even with standard chow, these mice are obese. Their microbes are different than their lean littermates: the obese ones have more Firmicutes and fewer Bacteroidetes. And guess what happened when the microbes from the ob/ob mice were inserted into the germ-free mice? They got fat. After two weeks, the recipients of the microbiota from the ob/ob mice extracted more calories from food and also showed a significantly greater fat gain than did mice that received the microbiota from lean mice.[32]

The microbiota in the ob/ob mice contain gene-encoding enzymes that break down otherwise indigestible dietary polysaccharides. They also found more end products of fermentation and fewer calories in the feces of the obese mice, a sign that microbes were wringing extra calories from food.[33]

Scientists of course were wondering about humans. They found a similar shift: obese people had more Firmicutes and fewer Bacteroidetes, two different phyla groups. Then they asked what would happen if the obese people lost weight. Would the microbes be affected?

Researchers put 12 obese people in a weight-loss program for a year, randomly assigning them to either a fat-restricted or carbohydrate-restricted low-calorie diet. After weight loss, the relative proportion of Bacteroidetes increased while Firmicutes declined. The changes correlated with weight loss, not the calorie level. Bacteroidetes were about 3 percent of the gut bacteria before dieting and about 15 percent after weight loss. It is unknown why obese people have more Firmicutes.[34]

But how, you may ask, would one go about getting some of those Bacteroidetes, the ones thinner people have?

A child in Africa eats differently than a child in Italy. Legumes and root vegetables are not to be confused with pasta and pizza. And as it turns out, the microbes inside their tummies are also different. In a recent comparison, researchers showed that children from a village in Burkina Faso had a higher proportion of Bacteroidetes (57% versus 22%) and a lower proportion of Firmicutes (27% versus 64%) than the Italians. The high-fiber diet, similar to that of early humans, favored the development of the polysaccharide-degrading

Bacteroidetes, suggested the study authors.[35] The microbes evolved alongside the food supply. We truly are what we eat. Or, more accurately, we are what we ate yesterday.

Gut microbes are good savers. Fat storage depends on an enzyme called lipoprotein lipase or LPL. If it is in short supply, the hoarding suffers. Something called fasting-induced adipocyte factor, or Fiaf, also inhibits the LPL supply. When Fiaf is abundant, less fat storage is taking place. But here is what happens when microbes jump into the fray: microbes reduce Fiaf, which results in more LPL, which in turn increases fat storage. As fat cells fill up, fat accumulates in other organs, leading to insulin resistance and a chronic inflammatory state.

Microbes regulate genes that deposit lipids in adipocytes. Changes are made in the expression of these genes.

Thus, gut microbes affect both sides of the energy balance equation: changing the harvest of energy from the diet as well as how energy is either burned or stowed away. Yet many questions remain. Among them:

1. What causes variation among individuals?

2. Are these a cause or effect of obesity?

3. Could small changes in calorie extraction result in meaningful differences in weight?

The answers are complex and full of twists.

For instance, microbes can encourage weight loss too. Specific microbes may get in the way of fat storage. Here are a few:

- *Lactobacillus gasseri BNR17* from human breast milk was given to rats on a high-carbohydrate diet. The percent increase in body weight and fat pad mass was lower in the BNR17 group.[36]

- In a Swedish study, another lactobacillus, *paracasei ssp paracasei F19 (F19)* decreased fat storage by altering lipoprotein lipase.[37]

- *Lactobacillus plantaraum* is another showing potential. In mice, it reduced fat cell size.[38]

But it is interesting that lactobacilli, part of the Firmicutes phyla, are often linked with obesity in published studies, unlike the above behavior.

- *Lactobacillus reuteri* was associated with obesity.[39]

- Lactobacillus can encourage growth as seen in chickens.[40]

- And infants fed with *Lactobacillus rhamnosus GG*-enriched formula grew better than those fed with regular formula.[41]

Then there are bifidobacteria, which are some of the most numerous probiotics in the gut. (They are not Bacteroidetes.)

- *Bifidobacterium spp.* was given to high fat diet-induced obese rats in a 2011 study. Results: reduced body and fat weights as well as other markers of a high-fat diet.[42]

These data suggest a promising new angle for treating obesity. But science is still sorting it out.

ANTIBIOTICS

What a breakthrough if bacteria could help in weight loss, right? Funny thing though, the food industry already knows all about weight management via microbiota manipulation. For weight gain. Antibiotics have been given to animals to increase weight for over fifty years. Initially the antibiotics were given to fight infection. But then the farmers noticed that the animals were heavier. And more profitable.

Avoparcin, widely used by farmers, is related to the more known antibiotic, vancomycin; it improves feed efficiency and increases weight gain in animals.

The industry knew antibiotics increased weight of their herds; they just didn't know why.

As far back as 1955, researchers knew that a few animals didn't gain weight on antibiotics. Animals bred to be germ-free didn't add weight when put on antibiotics. That was the first clue that microbes were involved.

How might antibiotics increase weight?

The exact way antibacterial agents improve growth is not well known, but several ideas have been floated:

- Nutrients are better absorbed because of a thinner small-intestinal epithelium.

- Nutrients are spared because of fewer competing microbes.

- Microbes that cause subclinical infections are reduced.

- Growth-depressing toxins from intestinal microflora are lower.

- Changes to enzyme activity improve food efficiency.[43]

Could Antibiotics Be Doing the Same Thing to Humans?

Researchers in France wondered the same thing.[44] They analyzed hospital records for adults referred for suspicion of infective endocarditis to La Timone Hospital in Marseille, France, over a five-year period. The antibiotic group received intravenous antibiotics for at least four weeks. The control group was the ones who proved negative and did not receive antibiotics. One year after hospital discharge, 16 of the 48 in the treated group gained a significant amount of weight. Only one in the control group did. Older males had a rougher time than most when it came to weight control: Three patients in the study were males, older than 65, and underwent vancomycin treatment without surgery. All of them became obese with weight increases of 44, 37, and 22 pounds respectively.

Other studies revealed weight gain with antibiotic use.

One study followed 11,532 children who had been exposed to antibiotics in the first two years of life. The infants given antibiotics in the first six months of life were 22 percent more likely to be overweight at age three than those given none.[45] A five-day course of antibiotics changes human gut microbes for up to four weeks with some still altered at six months, according to recent studies.[46]

And antibiotics in infants predict reduced numbers of

Bifidobacteria and Bacteroides, those associated with less obesity.[47]

Similar growth effects have been observed in children with long-term use of antibiotics, most notably the popular tetracycline, a phenomenon noticed since the 1950s.[48] While the studies were flawed in design and analysis, they largely showed the trend of weight gain in children on antibiotics, though much of this was a reversal of malnutrition. Certain antibiotics don't appear to cause weight gain; amoxicillin, for one, has not been associated with weight gain.

In this next section, we'll take a look at mental microbes—the kind you can't see under a microscope but infect your heart and brain in powerful ways.

SOCIAL CONTAGIONS

The old saying goes, if you want to know a person, look at their friends. This may also be true for weight.

Obesity can spread through social circles.

That was the suspicion of researchers at Harvard Medical School who set out to prove it by mining the Framingham survey—a leviathan trove of data describing the eating and health habits of thousands of people over decades. Here's a bit of backstory: The Framingham Heart Study began in 1948 with 5,209 people enrolled and then followed up with second and third generation cohorts; it continues today. All participants undergo physical examinations (including measurements of height and weight) and complete written questionnaires at regular intervals. The comprehensive data could possibly reveal if obesity spread from person to person.

The researchers evaluated the "densely interconnected social network of 12,067 people assessed repeatedly from 1971 to 2003." Using "longitudinal [over time] statistical [neighbor] models, [they] examined whether weight gain in one person was associated with weight gain in his or her friends, siblings, spouse, and neighbors."

This is what they found:

- A person's risk of becoming obese rose by nearly 60 percent if a friend of the same sex was obese. If the friend was a close one, the likelihood was much worse: 171 percent.

- Among pairs of adult siblings, if one sibling became obese, the chance that the other would become obese increased by 40 percent.

- If one spouse became obese, the likelihood that the other spouse would become obese increased by 37 percent.

- These effects were not seen among neighbors in the immediate geographic location, which helps rule out environmental factors. Social distance appears to be more important than geographic distance within these networks.

- Persons of the same sex had relatively greater influence on each other than those of the opposite sex. This includes friend pairs and sibling pairs.

- The spread of smoking cessation did not account for the spread of obesity in this network.[49]

Clearly, social distance appears to be more important than geographic distance within these networks.

A more recent study out of Brown University found that overweight and obese men and women, ages 18 to 25, were more likely to have romantic partners, best friends, casual friends, and family members who were also overweight.[50]

Surely people may be more at ease with people of similar characteristics. Some of the matchups may be due to what is termed *assortative mating*, which is when mates are "more similar than would be expected by chance alone."[51]

But as the Framingham analysis revealed, people are more likely to become obese if their friend, sibling, or spouse did. Behaviors leading to weight gain were contagious.

The spread of these behaviors may be straightforward:

Consider, your best friend treats you to a surprise birthday lunch at her favorite Brazilian *churrascaria*. Do you flip the stop card after ten servings of barbecued beef, lamb, pork, and chicken, or please her by going for all sixteen?

Or your mom spends all day making your favorites, lasagna and chocolate cake. How will you get away with eating only one portion without hurting her feelings?

But obesogenic social behaviors also surface from a less-conscious place. Eating quickly or excessive portions when our spouse does may hold a similar biological imperative as why we yawn when someone else yawns.

Psychologists in the last century have created various sophisticated theories for how people learn: from behavioral to cognitive to humanistic and more. Likely, a change in behavior to lose or gain weight involves all of them. People learn in different ways. A person may "learn" to love potato chips because they are front and center on the kitchen counter; or because a new boyfriend wants to share them; or because, "hey, life is too short."

Modeling is behavior or learning that comes from watching the actions and outcomes of others' behavior. We may find ourselves eating more or faster with a friend who does the same. A snacking husband may trigger our own trip to the kitchen.

Here's one example of how it works for good behavior. Men and women enrolled in a multicenter diabetes trial received either intensive behavioral weight-loss intervention or no weight counseling. Those in the first group lost more weight, which was no surprise. But their spouses, even though they had undergone no intervention, also lost more weight than the spouses in the second. They modeled their behavior. The researchers attributed some of the effect to healthier foods in the house.[52]

Friends and family are the inner circle, and it seems likely that their habits, both good and bad, will spread. But what about other groups such as church congregations? It seems religious groups may be sharing more than prayer and good intentions. Obesity is much more prevalent in some than others. As potluck suppers may be a common activity to all, something else is spreading the tendency to be obese. In the United States, Baptists have high rates, yet Mormons and Seventh-day Adventists have low rates. In fact, the first give little attention to weight, while the last two stress health and wellness with their flocks.[53]

Social pressures to conform at work may be even greater. We don't complain about excessive air-conditioning, enticing arrays of candy and sodas in the lunchroom, or even the stress of hours that stretch into late evening. All may contribute to obesity.

And what about social media circles? Could Mark and his billion plus friends have any impact on obesity? Many of Mark's friends are not shy about showing their bodies if not their body mass index. A photo parade of this magnitude should encourage a svelte populace, a cluster eager to look lean. That remains to be seen. What Facebook has done, however, is create a massive database eager for composting, not just in the advertising world but the scientific world as well. Scientists at Harvard Medical School did just that. Their 2013 study matched interests such as "outdoor fitness activities" and "television" with BMI statistics across the United States and also within New York City. As expected, the healthier activities matched up with less obesity. Online social media may be a new way to gauge real-world health outcomes for global populations worldwide.[54]

Another social change is worth considering. For instance, the stigma of being overweight may be lessening. As more people around the globe become obese, attitudes change.

Marketers in the fashion industry recognize the potential in targeting large women. Websites and magazines champion big, beautiful women. Modeling agencies hire overweight women.

While obesity may not be making a comeback as a twenty-first-century fashion accessory, there is precedent. In Africa, a continent still suffering with famine and malnutrition, thin is not the feminine ideal. It's easier to attract a mate if a woman has large hips and ample breasts for healthy fertility and childbearing. African-American women may view such cultural acceptance and even preference by males as an obstacle to healthy weights.

In most of history, obesity was a sign of wealth and affluence, and lean was left to the lower classes. These days, of course, you can never be too skinny or too rich, an anthem of upper classes everywhere, and—as obesity reaches epidemic numbers—increasingly beyond reach.

SOLUTIONS

In 2011, researcher Nikhil Dhurandhar in *Lancet Infectious Diseases*: "If infections contribute to human obesity, then entirely different prevention and treatment strategies and public health policies could be needed to address this subtype of the disorder. . . . Clinicians should be aware of infectobesity (obesity of infectious origin), and its potential importance in effective obesity management."[55] It appears that the gut microbiota together with host genotype and lifestyle contribute to obesity.

Although no substitute for proper diet and exercise, manipulation of the gut microbiota may represent a novel approach for treating obesity, one that has few adverse effects. Much work needs to be done, however; it will be critical to identify potential microbes from more than 1,000 different species in the gut, a daunting task.[56]

Until that time, we can do several things to get started at making our microbiome less likely to make fat.

1. Reduce unhealthy adenovirus exposure. Wash your hands, don't share cups with sick people, and spend more time outdoors.

2. Choose a vaginal birth for your child if at all possible. Encourage others to do the same. Breastfeed your baby. It is easy, sterile, and best for your child and you in countless ways. Don't give up too easily; crying is not always a sign of hunger. And don't accept free cans of formula at the hospital.

3. Strengthen your immune system with daily strenuous exercise as well as healthy food and long sleeps.

4. Avoid antibiotic use when possible. Why bring in the army when a bit of time and rest will heal? Antibiotics are lifesavers in certain cases, to be sure, but are overused and becoming less effective every day as they are more easily resisted by invaders.

5. Avoid foods from animals that have been raised on antibiotics. Be certain your free-range chickens are not plumped up with a lifetime, albeit brief, of pills.

6. Probiotics: it is too early to say which probiotic strains will help you lose weight or keep it off—there are simply too many and research has not advanced that

far yet. But expect this science to move very quickly. Governments are funding microbiome research in a big way. Private investors are opening their wallets for probiotic research too: anything that helps in the obesity battle will have huge payoff.

The bacteria mentioned in this chapter may turn out to be beneficial on their own, for a certain person or not at all. While we are waiting, it is best to eat from a variety of probiotic-rich foods: aged cheeses, yogurts, kefir, buttermilk, sauerkraut, kimchee, pickles, and many others. Supplements? Take one with several strains. For a full discussion on foods and supplements, visit www.ProbioticsNow.com.

7. Prebiotics: Those friendly bacteria we host expect to be fed. So what do they like to eat? Indigestible carbohydrates. Perhaps the best-known one is inulin, found in bananas, garlic, onions, wheat, asparagus, artichoke, and chicory root.

8. Phenols are also helpful. They act as antioxidants as well as inhibiting non-probiotic bacteria. You may have heard of some of them: phytoestrogens, flavonoids, tannins and polyphenols.

9. Read the excellent book on probiotics by microbiologist Gary B. Huffnagle called *The Probiotics Revolution*. In it he discusses everything about probiotics and prebiotics as well as the richest sources of phenols including: the skin of fruits and vegetables; the papery skin on nuts; juices like grape and cranberry that you can't see through; herbs and spices; breads made with starters; legumes—the darker the better; teas, especially green; and dark, bittersweet chocolates.[57]

And remember when we change habits, we also influence our friends.

The spread of obesity in social networks appears to be a factor in the epidemic. Yet social influence also suggests that this same force can slow the spread of obesity. Both good and bad behaviors can spread over a range of social ties. In the study mentioned earlier about the overweight and obese young people at Brown University who had more friends who were obese, it was also found that if some were intending to lose weight, a significant number of their friends did also. And in another, women, especially black women, were more likely to sign up if they had a social contact who had or was presently in the weight-control intervention. Best of all, they attended more group sessions, kept more journals, and lost more weight than participants without contacts.[58]

It is known that peer support makes people more successful at quitting smoking or losing weight. Weight Watchers is wildly successful in part because of this component. Positive health behaviors are contagious. Join a gym with a friend. Look silly lifting weights with a friend. Take a healthy-eating class with a friend. Encourage a friend; the pep talk will help you too. Sign up for a Twitter message for encouragement. Buy your friend a pedometer.

Researchers see a glimmer of hope in the fight against obesity. Medical and public health interventions might be more cost-effective than initially supposed, since health improvements in one person might spread to others.[59]

Going viral may be one answer to the obesity epidemic.

8

. . . .

FAT OR FLIGHT RESPONSE:
STRESS & OBESITY

Stress affects the human body in powerful ways.
Some of these make us gain weight.

Funny

DO YOU CRAVE A STALK OF CELERY WHEN stressed out? Of course not. Comfort food is rarely green unless it is mint ice cream cradled by a sweet waffle cone or a pickle slice buried inside a Big Mac. Regrettably, only something sugary or fatty seems to calm jittery nerves.

The relief offered by junk food appears straightforward: stress quashes self-control because we forget about arteries and abs when the world turns harsh. Why not reward ourselves for working hard in school or at the office? The reason that stress packs on the pounds always seemed fairly obvious: we eat foods that remind us of happier times—mom's chocolate cake, a corn dog at a carnival, or a bag of chips shared with friends. Comfort food was never about our stomachs but all in our heads.

Until now. New research confirms that these cravings are rooted in more than nostalgia. Yes, we are programmed deep in our protective protoplasm to seek sugary and fatty foods when the going gets tough. Our bodies drive us to eat comfort foods, rich in simple carbohydrates and dense fat, as part of the master plan called survival.

Chronic stress feeds obesity. And in light of obesity's gallop across the globe, our world may be more stressful now than any time in history.

HOW STRESS CAUSES OBESITY

Scientists at the Department of Animal Biology at the University of Pennsylvania know all about stress. Their laboratories, though tucked within a few bucolic acres of campus, are slammed up against one of the roughest zip codes in America, a neighborhood that struggles with crime. Nevertheless, deep inside the lab where the calm of measured scientific discovery reigns, stress is more likely to mean chronic variable stress (CVS), in bench work parlance. Stress is under the microscope. In one recent project, mice were subjected to various stresses: constant light, multiple cage changes, moves to another male's dirty cage, 15 minutes of physical restraint, novel noise using a white noise generator, and a new object such as a marble placed in the cage. Any similarities to typical college student life were merely coincidental.

The rodents were then given a choice of a high-fat, a high-protein, or a high-carbohydrate diet. The fatty diet was very popular. During chronic stress, "mice given free access to these diets . . . selected a greater proportion of their calories in the form of the high-fat diet compared to non-stressed [control] mice."[1] These beings were possibly recalling happier chow times to quell their discomfort, but most likely it was something else. Not unlike the many freshmen on Penn's campus (juggling the stresses of new social ties, academic expectations, and staying safe within the neighborhood "zone"), who eventually console themselves into bigger jeans, these mice were adapting to stress based on long-ingrained biological imperatives. And herein lies the rub: ancient mechanisms, life-saving when food was scarce, are still being deployed today in a sedentary world rife with rich foods and new psychosocial stresses.[2]

A binge on junk food will make life unpleasant in the long run when we must face up to uncomfortable weight gain. But in the short term, fatty food splurges assist in the immediate goal, which is to ease stress. That is the conclusion of one creative experiment, one that will make parents cringe. Researchers at the University of New South Wales in Australia separated mother rats from their litter for either a 15-minute period or for three hours a day.[3] Any parent who even fleetingly lost a child in a crowd will recognize the magnitude of the stress induced in these creatures. Then the rats were fed a menu of either plain or high-fat food after which "anxiety and depression-like behaviors [were] assessed by elevated plus maze (EPM) and forced swim (FST) tests." Results? Those on fatty chow showed less mental pain.[4] These and similar findings suggest we are doubly doomed: not only does stress direct us to choose the Big Mac, but the good feelings right afterward reinforce the choice of junk food. So a part of the obesity problem is that eating comfort foods works: we feel better, at least until our skinny jeans strangle our thighs.

We all know people who actually eat less when upset or anxious. It is true that while 40 percent of people eat more when stressed, the same percentage will eat less. Those in the upper range of normal or overweight are more likely to eat when stressed. But everyone when stressed, regardless of whether they eat more or fewer total calories, favors fatty and sugary foods.[5] So, even if only a few billion on the planet are wired to eat more when stressed, it could explain some of the obesity epidemic.

But let's back up for a minute, to a pre-denim era, when fashion meant woolly mammoth fur in the winter and palm fronds in the summer.

Imagine a Neanderthal woman facing a hungry lion. Her stress reaction is called "fight-or-flight" because a rush of hormones jumpstarts the mind and body into quick action. It goes like this:

- The adrenal glands secrete epinephrine and cortisol. Epinephrine releases and cortisol boosts a torrent of glucose, supplying quick energy to large muscles, the heart, and the brain.

- Epinephrine and cortisol tighten the arteries as epinephrine speeds the heart rate, pumping blood faster.

- Neanderthal woman decides to fight or flee.

Modern stressors may not be as dramatic as wild animals of primeval times. But they are pervasive and often relentless, creating chronic stress, which can be deadlier than the single episode to which our body's defense mechanisms are better suited. In today's world, the stress response can be elicited by virtual or social pressures like an email message with a new deadline or a Facebook slight from an old boyfriend. Such psychosocial stresses may linger and, most important, require little energy: sitting and worrying are more likely than fighting or fleeing.

And when stress hangs on, cortisol and other players such as leptin and neuropeptide Y (NPY) stay on high alert, causing big problems. Here are ten of them:

Blood Sugar Rises

Cortisol boosts blood sugar during emergencies to drum up needed energy. For an in-depth explanation, read Dina Aronson's excellent article "Cortisol—Its Role in Stress, Inflammation, and Indications for Diet Therapy" in *Today's Dietitian* online.[6]

Here's the quick version of how cortisol preps the body for "fight or flight":

- The liver makes new glucose (or blood sugar).

- Glucose stays in blood, ready for action instead of going to storage in cells.

- These cells send signals to the brain—"Where's my lunch?"

- End result: the appetite police in the brain tell us to eat.

Abdominal Fat Increases

Cortisol plucks fatty acids from fat cells in thighs and hips and shuttles them closer to the action in the abdomen.

Transferring energy reserves from the side flanks to the front lines makes survival sense; the move makes our bodies more battle ready. But this strategy is not without risk. This visceral fat has been referred to as "toxic fat," because of strong links to heart attacks and strokes. Also, visceral fat has lots of cortisol receptors, thus laying out the welcome mat for marauding stress hormones. Once inside, cortisol excites lipoprotein lipase, which encourages even more fat deposits. And the circus continues as more cortisol is converted from cortisone. Clearly fat is a not just a blob of quiet tissue but a dynamic endocrine organ, a distinction discerned only in the last decade.

Cravings for High-Calorie Foods

Cortisol calls for backup. It goes right to the top—the hypothalamus in the brain, where signals are sent to eat more high-calorie foods. When cortisol is high, appetite follows. There is a link between cortisol levels and calorie intake in some women.[7]

Appetite Stimulants Continue Receiving Signals

Neuropeptide Y (NPY) is released from sympathetic nervous system fibers, what we call nerves, during times of extreme stress. NPY upends the normal fat-making process, especially if excess cortisol is around to encourage it: abdominal fat cells increase in both number (by converting pre-adipocytes into mature fat cells) and size (by filling up with lipids). NPY stimulates mouse and human fat growth, and cortisol is behind it.[8]

Leptin Resistance Ensues

Leptin kills appetite. Leptin was going to save us from the obesity epidemic, but it didn't work out that way: obese people don't respond to supplemental leptin—because they have plenty. Much as type 2 diabetics are resistant to insulin, obese people are resistant to the leptin swimming through their bodies.[9] In fact, circulating leptin is directly proportional to the amount of fat in the body. And when stress hormones join the mix, leptin resistance worsens. This means big appetite.

Sex Hormones Decline

Beyond the obvious, sex hormones are helpful in another way: they mobilize fat stores. When they decline, fat metabolism changes. For example, when patients undergo anti-androgenic therapies for polycystic ovary syndrome or prostate cancer, they gain weight. Chronic stress also subdues these hormones.

Hypothalamic-Pituitary-Adrenal Axis (HPA) Changes

Addiction studies suggest that the brain circuitry involved in reward is also a key player in stress-induced food intake. At the

University of California, San Francisco, researchers found that when restrained rats ingested comfort foods, their actual stress to the same restraints was lowered. How did they know this? The researchers observed reduced activity in the hypothalamic-pituitary-adrenal (HPA), an axis critical to mobilizing energy sources under stress.[10]

Chronic stress leads to eating comfort foods, which leads to abdominal fat, which dampens the HPA response, which means less cortisol. Voilà. Rutgers University scientists tested this theory in 59 young women. The high-stress group had higher BMIs, rounder abdomens, and more emotional eating. They also showed blunted cortisol in response to a lab stressor.[11]

In a lab in 2013 at the University of California, Davis, 41 women were subjected to either a social stress test or a nature movie. Then they were "invited to a buffet [of both] low- and high-calorie snacks." The women who reported more chronic stress (but also responded with less cortisol to the acute stress test) ate more calories from chocolate cake. They also had more total fat, regional fat, and negative mood with stress.[12]

Stress and comfort foods couple in the memory, noted researcher Mary F. Dallman in *Trends in Endocrinology & Metabolism*. That matchup will be remembered and can turn into a habit that requires little conscious thought. The comfort food can be used again and again to soothe stress, a reward path where compulsive eating takes hold. There are two problems with this. First, the extra calories will settle in the abdomen, a dangerous spot because of stress hormones, and second, once comforted, the individual doesn't confront the stressor. Dallman wrote that "Once stress-induced feeding becomes habitual, the problem-solver, executive part of the prefrontal cortex may no longer be actively engaged in the outcome; 'comfort food' intake may become a reflex."[13]

Eighty healthy students at Ruhr University Bochum in Germany took part in a study that asked if stress interfered with "goal-directed actions." Some of the students were made to immerse a hand in ice water for three minutes. Blood pressure, salivary cortisol, and observation confirmed stress. Sure enough, a series of tests led the scientists to conclude that stress acted "as a switch between 'cognitive' and 'habit' learning systems."[14]

The prefrontal cortex is the part of the brain most sensitive to stress. "Even quite mild acute uncontrollable stress can cause a rapid and dramatic loss of prefrontal cognitive abilities, and more prolonged stress exposure causes architectural changes in prefrontal dendrites," wrote Yale researcher Amy Arnsten.[15]

While habit is a vital to learning—think about driving a car—cognitive ability to predict and direct outcomes is crucial. But stress prefers habits.

This makes compulsive eating more likely the next time a cortisol-pumping episode strikes.

Brain Damage

Chronic stress can damage the brain. It changes delicate structure and function, which leads to cognitive and mood disturbances. "The hippocampus . . . important in learning and memory, is particularly sensitive to chronic stress and to [cortisol]."[16] It shrinks. Magnetic resonance imaging (MRI) showed a 3 percent drop in hippocampal volume in chronically restrained rats.[17] Other studies on "neuroticized" rats and monkeys revealed similar atrophy on dissection. It is intriguing how neuroticization was induced: rats were subjected to 15 minutes daily of electro-pain irritation accompanied by four hours daily of white noise over a total period of three weeks. (White noise is a random signal of every frequency in the sound spectrum).

Diabetes Develops

In 2010, a gene that ties stress to diabetes was identified. A research team at the Weizmann Institute Neurobiology Department in Israel found that change in a single gene could cause mice to exhibit anxiety and develop diabetic symptoms. They suspected Urocortin-3 (Ucn3) was responsible. This protein helps regulate the stress response. Higher levels in certain parts of the mouse brain led to anxiety and changes in metabolism; mice burned more carbohydrates and fewer fatty acids as metabolic rates sped up. There were signs of type 2 diabetes: A drop in muscle sensitivity to insulin, which delayed sugar uptake by the cells, resulting in raised sugar levels in the blood.[18]

177

Ghrelin Climbs

Ghrelin stands alone as the only known hormone that stimulates appetite rapidly. Recent research has highlighted relationships between ghrelin, stress, and lifestyle factors: Researchers at the University of Southwestern Texas Medical Center found in animal studies that stress can cause ghrelin levels to rise—thus stimulating appetite—and that ghrelin has a function in changing mood.[19]

Wow. Stress isn't all in our heads.

The breadth of adaptation to chronic stress—and these are just the ones we know—is humbling. The living organism, whether man, mouse, or single-celled amoeba, adapts to its stressful environment. Marvel at the ten above mentioned ways the human body rallies to protect itself: the intricate dance of molecules, hormones, enzymes, axes, and yet undiscovered players is enough to shake an atheist's credo.

MODERN STRESS IS DIFFERENT

Be thankful, for survival's sake, that we have these adaptations when danger really strikes. But many modern stresses only mimic danger. How truly dangerous is that traffic jam? Or your boss's bad attitude? Yet even in psychosocial pseudo-stressful scenarios, stress conspires to save energy and make us fat. Be it acute or chronic, real or imagined, stress can make us fat.

The logic: If stress causes weight gain, it follows that our *epidemic of obesity means that the world is more stressful than it was in the past.* Surely this is not true, is it? Is today's world as anxiety-fraught as life was for a caveman, who never knew when the next saber-toothed tiger would invite itself to dinner? Is it as stressful as famines, world wars, or the plague?

In a word, yes. Technology has released many of us from certain pressures, such as wondering from where our next meal will come or how we will heat the cabin in a brutal winter. But life today antagonizes with small stressors like no other time in history: long commutes, college applications, colonoscopies, job insecurity, over-medicated kids, and outliving our money are just the beginning. Even incessant cell phone beeps add an annoying layer.

We experience more of a specific type of stress today, more than all the people in all of history; we have more of the stress called chronic stress. Our bodies were designed for confronting and acting on acute or isolated stresses: the rabid dog, the brewing storm, or in a more relevant example, any podium with our name on it. As we saw in the beginning of this chapter, chronic or repeated stress keeps cortisol and insulin levels elevated; this pair along with their compatriots destroy the hum in our hummers. Let's start by looking at what exactly in our modern, comfortable lives underwrites chronic stress.

No Downtime

Was "24/7" even a concept that existed before the new millennium? In fact, nine-to-five was long the workplace standard, except of course for the unlucky medical residents and night shift workers. Stimulation never lets up now: longer hours at work, cell phones connecting us all the time, hundreds of television channels, Facebook, Twitter, iPads, Kindles, and the rest of the constantly upgraded landscape of technology. Shift workers are at particular risk. Scientists at the Stress Research Institute in Stockholm wrote:

> Compared to individuals who work during the day, shift workers are at higher risk of a range of metabolic disorders and diseases (e.g., obesity, cardiovascular disease, peptic ulcers, gastrointestinal problems, failure to control blood sugar levels, and metabolic syndrome). At least some of these complaints may be linked to the quality of the diet and irregular timing of eating; however, other factors that affect metabolism are likely to play a part, including psychosocial stress, disrupted circadian rhythms, sleep debt, physical inactivity, and insufficient time for rest and revitalization.[20]

More Perceived Threats

Remember, stress is a perceived threat, not a measure of the actual threat. We are scared of home invasions, terrorist attacks, snake bites, bird flu, skin cancer, biological terrorism, and countless tales of horror and impending doom dug up and sensationalized by the 24-hour news stations. In *Bowling for Columbine*, a documentary about societal violence, Michael Moore makes the point that news coverage is sowing fear and distrust across America.

And here is a totally fresh condition named cyberchondria: anxiety caused by Googling or Binging health symptoms. It's not too difficult to make the leap from irregular mole to death by malignant melanoma when our village is now the world and someone somewhere is sick and blogging about it.

Expectations Have Changed

In modern times, at least in developed countries, we are so accustomed to good fortune that when tragedy strikes, we ask, "Why me?" More than most people in history, I suspect, we expect life to be happy—though those Roman nobles sure looked to be having some fun. As recently as the 1800s, mothers in western cultures stayed emotionally aloof from their newborns; too many babies died in the first few years. Today, we assume our children will outlive us; in the same optimistic vein, we expect our doctors will cure us and our employers will pay us enough for vacations and new bathrooms. People expect if they play by the rules, life will be good to them. But it doesn't work like that. Life brings setbacks, loss, and suffering. That's life and it's stressful.

Standards Have Changed

On a lighter yet potentially more troubling note, look at the pressure today to look good or be rich. Media have made us aware of others' lives though sugarcoated Photoshopped lenses. Of course, they want beautiful people on their pages or websites. Who doesn't steal a guilty peek at *People Magazine* in the dentist's waiting room? You only have to look at rates of plastic surgery to see that standards and norms are being transformed rapidly. The stress of looking good today has amplified: photo shoots on Facebook, tagging on Facebook, everybody marketing themselves as a brand. Could teeth be any whiter or straighter? Could breasts be any higher or rounder? Whole swaths of the planet—California and Brazil in particular— have older women who look like teenagers with smooth skin, wide eyes, and other surgical enhancements.

Keeping up with the Joneses has never been more bruising, to body or soul. The stress is amplified for people in poor countries who now have front-row seats via television at a banquet they cannot share.

Change Is Nonstop

Even good things can be stressful if there are too many of them.

Perhaps you recall a published list of life events that assigned stress points to your life and when you went above a certain number: Of course! You have a right to be stressed out! Marriage, a new job, a new house, and even a new baby—all positive things—added points. True, we may be having fewer babies but definitely, current times have brought serial marriages as well as serial jobs with more relocations.

Were our bodies meant for air travel, speeding across time zones, disrupting circadian rhythms? Likely not, though young people seem to handle it better than older ones. A clever experiment from the University of Virginia tested just how well mice adapt to a series of light-cycle changes that simulated time zone hopping. It turns out the forward shift (equivalent of going west to east or the red eye flight from New York to London) was tougher than the reverse. The researchers found that the younger mice survived whereas only 47 percent of the older ones lived for their hypothetical return flight across the pond.[21]

Less Balance

This may be the true repetitive stress injury—anything in excess or at the exclusion of other activities is not healthy. I once wrote a newspaper article about stress and stay-at-home mothers versus working mothers, and guess who came out saner in the research and interviews? It was the women with balanced lives, the ones who "had it all" even if that meant juggling careers and motherhood. That argument, with men and women today sharing roles, jobs, and childcare, should bode well on the "stress-ometer." Yet with workaholic habits where employers expect more and more while cutting pensions, health benefits, and job security, tensions are sure to rise.

Less power

These professions are often cited as stressful:

- Inner City High School Teacher
- Police Officer
- Miner
- Air Traffic Controller
- Medical Intern
- Stockbroker
- Journalist
- Customer Service Worker
- Secretary
- Waiter

What do most of these professions have in common? Doing the job well depends on the cooperation of others. The medical intern is not only working long hours but can potentially hurt someone with a wrong decision. Even if all the right decisions are made, patients still die. In that regard, they are powerless to determine many outcomes. And many of these careers attract sensitive people, those who will suffer if their services are not well received. Burnout is inevitable.

Power struggles are hardly new. Each of the twelve apostles jostled for position next to Jesus. Governments are overthrown weekly it seems. Our awareness of humans with high status has grown exponentially. No longer do we compare our positions in the local group, but we are forced to measure up to Hollywood faces and Wall Street bank accounts. It is harder to feel good when the whole world is our tribe.

Status impacts appetite.

Scientists at the Yerkes National Primate Research Center at Emory University in Atlanta tested the theory with rhesus macaques. The socially subordinate females consumed more of both the low-fat diet and the high-fat diet than the dominant females throughout a 24-hour period. And while the outranked animals took to nighttime binging, the dominant females only ate during the daytime hours.

This feeding behavior showed up as an increase in fat-derived hormones and weight gain in the lower ranks.[22]

In a paper titled "Environmental Contributions to the Obesity Epidemic," the authors summarized biological responses in the subordinate or less powerful: "In primates, subordinate individuals have a different neuro-immune-endocrine fingerprint: they are relatively hypercortisolemic, have an increased NPY release, an enhanced appetite, leptin resistance, and central fat deposition."[23]

A similar response to stress was found in a long-term British survey called the Whitehall II Study. More than 8,000 adults were screened over ten-year periods. Lower occupational position predicted adverse changes in waist circumference, BMIs, and other metabolic markers.[24]

And using civil service employment grade and measures of work stress, researchers found that employees with chronic work stress were 50 percent more likely to be obese than those without.[25]

In other words, lack of power corrupts too.

One more disturbing observation is this: underlings in animal trials eked out more calories from the same chow. Gram for gram, dominant animals, arrogant in their survival skills perhaps, metabolized food less efficiently.[26] What does this tell us? Perhaps obese people aren't eating as much as others assume; their metabolisms are different.

Take a look at several scenarios that serve as uniquely modern stresses.

Having a sick child is stressful; having a child diagnosed with cancer is another type of stress entirely, the unthinkable kind. The Children's Hospital of Pittsburgh is a first-rate facility that treats thousands of these young patients yearly. And because of the generous nature of the parents who bring their children here, researchers were able to enroll enough parents to study how the stress of such a diagnosis would have on their weight. Participants consisted of 49 parents of pediatric cancer patients and 49 parents of healthy children. Parents with children diagnosed with cancer reported less physical activity, more sedentary behavior, and lower caloric intake than parents with healthy children. At the end of three months, the parents of children with cancer had gained more weight than parents of healthy children. Interestingly, the most dramatic difference in weight-related behavior between the two sets of parents was with physical activity rather than diet.[27] However, as was seen above, stressed subordinates in animal trials gained more weight than the unstressed dominants from the same amount of chow.[28] Even if they had been kings and queens, these parents would have felt powerless.

Cancer screenings save lives. But they also add untold stress and anxiety to life. Pap smears, mammograms, colonoscopies, and prostate-antigens all represent the challenges of health care in the twenty-first century. Millions of tests are finding abnormalities that may disappear in time or take a lifetime to kill. The angst provoked by waiting for test results is a thoroughly modern stress. The toll continues even if it was a false-positive, a common occurrence. Danish researchers found that six months after false-positive results on a mammogram, women had distress as high as those with breast cancer. Anxiety over the cancer scare still lingered three years later.[29]

Not far from the Children's Hospital in the lively Oakland section of Pittsburgh is Carnegie Mellon University, where research on stress is coming up with some interesting data. Psychologist Sheldon Cohen and his team at the Laboratory for the Study of Stress, Immunity and Disease found that women and those with lower income and less education were more stressed. But as people aged, stress lessened.[30] Cohen has looked at stress from many angles and three decades ago was wondering what noise did to health. He found that noise caused a generalized stress reaction, causing hormonal jumps and higher blood pressure.[31]

And across the ocean, researchers at the Federal Environmental Agency in Berlin, Germany, reviewed papers from the past three decades and reported that the biggest echo "of chronic noise exposure seems to be the development of hypercortisolism." Traffic noise caused surges of cortisol even when people were sleeping; this persisted if the noise was repeated consistently.[32]

Noise is a recent invention: the industrial revolution brought factories, jackhammers, guns, washing machines, vacuum cleaners, and automobile traffic. To experience a city without traffic din, travel to Venice, Italy, and ride a gondola to your hotel. The quiet is blissful. The gentle lapping of water replaces the traffic noises. Yes, manufactured noise is another distinctly modern stress.

And here's another. Driving, most people will concede, can be stressful. Driving in Cairo, Egypt, where I have lived for six years, is not unlike carnival bumper cars, with barnyard animals as combatants. There are terrible drivers on every asphalt and gravel stretch of the planet—Mexico City and Boston have more than their share—but Egyptians, who are some of the kindest people on the planet, win the prize with their disdain for licenses, laws, headlights, turn signals, and brakes. Surviving the erratic driving amid goats, potholes, and exhaust fumes can usually be managed with patience and defensive driving. But here's the most stressful part of the experience: the constant bleating of the car horns. In Egypt, horns substitute for brakes and turn signals; they announce, "Watch out—here I come." There is emerging evidence of an association between road traffic and aircraft noise and health problems. Cars and planes are not going away, and neither is the noise.

Finally, there is post-traumatic stress; the world has always had it but we didn't label it. World War II was every bit as traumatic as conflicts in Iraq and Afghanistan except now we have a name for the predictable fallout to soldiers' psyches. In fact, behavior as usual may indicate an aberrant response in these cases. When these young people try to resume their civilian lives, many can't do it. Suicides are on the rise. Recent research from the Centre for Military and Veterans' Health at the University of Adelaide in Australia points to a litany of physical problems as well stemming from trauma: "PTSD is associated with a significant body of physical morbidity in the form of chronic musculoskeletal pain, hypertension, hyperlipidemia, obesity and cardiovascular disease. This increasing body of literature suggests that the effects of traumatic stress need to be considered as a major environmental challenge that places individual's physical and psychological health equally at risk."[33] Actually, overweight and obesity rates among United States veterans are higher than already high rates in the general population, with the highest rates among veterans with PTSD.[34]

Trauma takes all forms, not just the horrific scale of war. Trauma can be anything inducing painful memories and parallel stress responses: death of a loved one, bullying in childhood, a car accident, or anything perceived as traumatic.

People respond differently to stress. Thus the amount of cortisol secreted in response to stress varies among individuals. Healthy women who react to stress with high levels of cortisol secretion also tend to eat more when under stress than women who secrete less. Furthermore, women with most of their stored fat in the abdominal area have higher cortisol levels and report more lifestyle stress than women who are apt to store fat in their hips.[35]

SOLUTIONS

Stress demands a response. The problem with using food for comfort, in addition to obesity, is that we are avoiding the problem. Whether you are worried about money, a child, or a job, seek help from a good friend or a counselor. Also, step up and help when others are stuck.

Just knowing that our bodies may urge us to eat more when under siege is helpful. We can counteract those orders:

Breathe. Take a deep breath, exhale, repeat, then do it again. This will slow the rapid heart rate.

Pray. Meditate. As hard as it may be to sit still and rest your busy mind, prayer and meditation salve the spirit. And research shows the brain chemistry and actual structure changes as practice grows. The advent of sophisticated brain imaging has proven how potent these techniques can be. For example, "putting feelings into words (affect labeling) . . . diminished the response of the amygdala and [other] regions [of the brain] to negative emotional images."[36] And this may be the best news of all: the damage done by stress to our brain structure and function can be reversed.[37]

Neuroplasticity is a remarkable discovery that offers hope across the spectrum of mental health. Because comfort food does actually soothe and then becomes a harmful habit for the stressed brain, mindful thinking and meditation are required to bring the process back under the control of the prefrontal cortex.

Mindfulness training should be taught in schools and communities. Do as the Dalai Lama says, "I find hope in the darkest of days, and focus in the brightest. I do not judge the universe."

Yoga. Hypnosis. Acupuncture.

Balance. Do it all. Work, swim, ride a bike, visit a friend. Maybe you just need a break.

Put the problem in perspective. In 1996, Richard Carlson published a little book that sold in a big way. *Don't Sweat the Small Stuff—and it's all small stuff* deserves a spot next to your bed, desk, or wherever you need to destress.[38]

Limit computer time. Read a book at the park, watch a movie in a theater, and pay a bill in person.

Choose your companions. Surround yourself with positive people.

Take control of your life. Break out of routines that no one is really imposing on you, or even if they are. Forget status. Nobody really cares about the size of your house, your paycheck, or your body; they are too busy thinking about their own.

If the stressor is big, such as a terminal illness, stress responses are more than justified. But still you must manage them. Waiting for results of a cancer screen? Psychologists say people handle it differently. Some imagine the worst and then anything less is a relief. Others keep busy to distract a worried mind.

Write in a journal or diary, advises Mary F. Dallman. Writing requires activity of the thinking brain, the prefrontal cortex, and makes people confront issues. It also pulls you back from the cloud of anxiety, she said, into the moment. "NOW is rarely catastrophic, things are not so bad in the moment of writing, and some clarity may be gained,"[39] she said. An excellent guide was written by researcher James W. Pennebaker, *Writing to Heal: A Guided Journal for Recovering from Trauma and Emotional Upheaval.* Pennebaker's pioneering work showed that writing can benefit those experiencing all types of trauma, from first year at college to terminal illness.[40]

Count your blessings. Think of less-fortunate people instead of celebrities on television. In fact, a way to fight depression according to self-help books is to help someone. It works: not only do we like ourselves better because we are "good" but we compare our lives favorably to the persons we are helping. In other words, we have a new clan, one in which we shine, one in which we have moved up in the hierarchy. While this may sound like a perversion of good, it yields good results for everyone involved.

Make a plan to solve the problem or prevent the thing you're worried about. Begin it. Confucius said, "A journey of a thousand miles begins with one step." In 1995, Anne Lamott wrote a thoughtful memoir on life and writing and loss. Her story is this: When she was a young girl, Anne had to do a term paper on birds of North America but was frustrated at how to begin. Her father's advice to her became the title of her book: *Bird by Bird*.[41] It's a useful mantra for overwhelming situations even if homework in your life is a distant memory.

Eat Well

When *Managing Your Mind & Mood Through Food* was published in 1988, I was captivated.[42] Here was a revolutionary theory in the staid nutrition field: food could make us happy, relaxed, energetic, or focused. I already knew that eating too much chocolate cake could make me depressed. Yet author Judith Wurtman, Massachusetts Institute of Technology researcher and scientific heavyweight, was purporting all sorts of crazy stuff: she was spinning mealtime like a mood ring. As the decades have sped by, her book has only garnered more acceptance. Wurtman writes that the right food at the right time in the right amount is as effective as a tranquilizer (quaint term for Valium and its ilk) for the acute stresses of daily life.

Carbohydrates work best, she says, and here's why: they raise the levels of an amino acid called tryptophan, which in turn boosts serotonin, a compound that calms us. A big wedge of chocolate cake is not advised here; a small bran muffin with honey perhaps or fresh fruit with creamy yogurt is much better.[43]

Protein, on the other hand, has the opposite immediate effect: it keeps us awake and alert. Whisk up an omelet for your child on the morning before a big test; in addition to whites, which are full of protein, yolks are rich in choline, another plus for enriching memory. Or try a berry smoothie fortified with tofu. Even if they don't know all the answers, those kids won't be snoozing. And just eating breakfast regularly predicted higher scores on IQ tests in Chinese kindergartners in research done at the University of Pennsylvania School of Nursing. Don't skip it.[44]

Chronic stress—the kind that leads to obesity—and its management take more planning. A nutritious diet can counteract the impact of stress by shoring up the immune system, decreasing inflammation, and lowering blood pressure.

Here are some helpful guidelines:

- Caffeine, alcohol, trans fats, and saturated fats should be avoided to minimize inflammation.

- Dark chocolate has flavonoids. Make sure it has 70 percent or more cacao.

- Tea, especially chamomile, fights anxiety.

- Oatmeal is a perfect carbohydrate to boost the calming brain chemical serotonin because it's high in fiber and won't mess with blood sugar levels. Whole grain crackers and rice cakes also work well.

- Omega-3 fatty acids help reduce stress. It is widely accepted that the ratio of Q6:Q3 in the daily diet should be in balance—the optimum ratio and recommendations vary from country to country with Japan advising 2:1 and Sweden advising 5:1. The average American diet, which is low in fish, is estimated to be 8:1 to 12:1 with some as high as 25:1.

- Though all nuts are probably helpful to some extent, walnuts are the darlings right now. Preliminary analyses suggest walnuts can alter stress signals. It appears that linolenic acid is effective in lowering stress signals.

- Probiotics. These helpful bacteria can change mood. One recent study out of Ireland used the probiotic *Bifidobacterium infantis* with rats that were then placed in stressful situations. The study concluded, "Probiotic treatment resulted in normalization of the immune response, reversal of behavioral deficits, and restoration of hormone concentrations in the brainstem."[45] Eat yogurt, aged cheeses, and other cultured foods.

- Aromatherapy is gaining scientific support. Sweet

orange scents calmed anxiety in humans in a study from Brazil.[46]

- And the quickest way to dissolve stress? Move. Exercise is a magic bullet for stress. Here's why:

The stress response demands a physical response. This made more sense when physical aggression was the major stress in ancient times. Danger made us fight or flee; both meant movement. Today, psychosocial stresses from traffic, medical tests, and excessive demands excite these same hormones though we are rarely forced to outrun an angry boss. The energy mobilized by modern stress is not used. Instead it is stored as fat. A slew of other metabolic disturbances ensue as was mentioned at the beginning of this chapter.

Because the stress response is a neuroendocrine tool that occurs in expectation of movement, exercise should be the natural answer to stress. It works. Numerous studies confirm the vast benefits of exercise in stress: for preventing or for relieving and for both physical and mental problems.[47]

But what to do when stress escalates into anxiety or panic attacks? After exhausting all the techniques mentioned above, from proper eating to mediation to vigorous exercise, try this: Challenge the way you are thinking. Are you willing to bet something valuable that your fear will come true? This works well, especially when all other anxiety relievers short of medication have failed. Betting puts the odds of something happening into plain terms. We are forced to see the facts and tune out all the neurotic voices and racing thoughts. We can learn a lot from people who don't seem to have stress, who sail through life without dwelling on every setback. Resilience can be learned.

And in closing, this last encouraging note: Habits of thinking need not be forever.

"One of the most significant findings in psychology in the last twenty years is that individuals can choose the way they think," writes Martin Seligman, author of *Learned Optimism*.[48] This University of Pennsylvania researcher and father of positive psychology decided that modern psychology spent far too much time studying the origins of deviant behavior and not enough analyzing what makes happy people tick.

Indeed, positive psychology has a lot to teach us about handling stress. Pills may be quicker, but then of course you need pills. Positive psychology weaves all the methods listed above with cognitive therapy. Study it, practice it, prioritize it, and teach it to your children; it's every bit as important as algebra. And when we learn to limit chronic stress, not only will life be happier but we can also say good-bye to metabolisms fighting to put on extra pounds of fat. And that alone makes me feel better.

9

· · · ·

PUMPED UP: FOOD ADDITIVES & OBESITY

Hormones and antibiotics are two additives given to the animals we eat. Along with hundreds in other foods, we get more than our healthy share.

NOT LONG AGO WHILE ENJOYING A TRACTOR ride amid green pastures and big skies of a Pennsylvania spring, I came across the youngest member of the dairy farm I was visiting: a newborn calf.

The sight of an animal up on its four legs within minutes of leaving the birth canal is magical, one that makes our own species look lazy in comparison. Humans coddle their offspring for decades and often feed them pretty poorly. But animals at this small family farm in Forks Township, Pennsylvania, eat well; they benefit from a precision diet including eight strains of probiotics sprinkled in their feed.

Owner Layne Klein prefers probiotics to antibiotics, which he only uses as a last resort as when a cow gets an infection called mastitis. Such prudence is a rarity these days, especially on big industrial farms, which produce the bulk of American meat and dairy foods.

Antibiotics—routinely given to add weight—are only the beginning. Ine most steps along the way, from feedlot to factory to supermarket to dinner table and even when stored as leftovers, our food is exposed to potentially harmful chemicals. Many of these were introduced in the last three decades when not so coincidentally obesity rates have exploded.

The chemicals are diverse: antibiotics and growth hormones in animal feed; fungicides and pesticides on produce; preservatives, colorants, and flavor enhancers in processing; plastic in packaging as well as reheating and serving containers of food and beverages. Some are added by design while others latch on or leach out unintentionally.

And they are abundant: More than 60 pounds of corn sweeteners, mostly high-fructose corn syrup, were produced for every person in the United States in 2011.[1]

It must be stressed that *chemical* is not a dirty word. All matter—humans and rocks included—is a conflagration of chemicals. Certain chemicals in our food help us by killing harmful pathogens. Others prevent spoilage. But some are dangerous; many have been banned because of their links to cancer and other diseases. And know this: something as natural as salt from a shaker can be more harmful than a synthetic chemical cooked up in a lab. Each one has its own personality.

Some like to fatten us up. Many are obesogens. This means that chemicals disturb normal hormonal systems and can lead to weight gain. Obesogens are very clever in their modus operandi: they mimic natural hormones, persuade stem cells to become fat cells, and perhaps even change genes.

Food should not be so complicated. As you read on, you will see that the twenty-first-century food supply is anything but simple. It is a chemically leavened, synthetically enhanced multibillion dollar business propelled by lobbyists and lax government enforcement.

Technology feeds more people at lower cost—a miracle for the planet. But all the scientific brilliance coupled with profit motives has had an unintended result: we eat too much and store too much fat. Now for the first time since man appeared a half million years ago, obesity is as big a problem as hunger.

Take a look at how obesogens operate after wheedling their way into three different stages of the food supply.

Could it be from antibiotics mixed in chicken feed? Or possibly the growth hormones implanted in cattle? Or the high-fructose corn syrup in soda or the monosodium glutamate in noodle soups or the chemicals leaking into foods from plastic storage containers?

There are many suspects.

ANTIBIOTICS

Antibiotics are first in the lineup. The wonder drugs of the twentieth century, antibiotics rushed in with the discovery of penicillin. Since then, millions of lives have been saved from serious infections. It may come as a surprise then to learn that the overwhelming majority of antibiotics in the United States—nearly 80 percent—are sold for use in food animals, not humans, according to former FDA-commissioner David A. Kessler writing in the *New York Times* in 2013.[2]

Low-dose antibiotics are given to animals to prevent infection (cows, pigs, and chickens live in tight quarters) and to add weight—a profitable practice when a sirloin steak commands a premium price per pound.

But too many antibiotics means the bacteria learn to fight back; they become drug-resistant bacteria, staying a beat ahead of our drug pipeline.

In a 2011 news release, Margaret Chan, WHO Director-General is quoted as saying, "The world is on the brink of losing these miracle cures in the absence of urgent corrective and protective actions, the world is heading towards a post-antibiotic era, in which many common infections will no longer have a cure and, once again, kill unabated."[3]

United States policy is under scrutiny.

"With the occasional exception, like cephalosporins," wrote Dr. Robert S. Lawrence of Johns Hopkins Bloomberg School of Public Health in *The Atlantic* magazine, "[the] FDA has failed for decades to take meaningful action on the misuse of antibiotics in food animal production—misuse that directly contributes to the selection of antibiotic-resistant bacteria and compromises our ability to treat bacterial infections."[4]

Recently, the FDA has asked that antibiotics be available for animals only by prescription from veterinarians. Whether a gatekeeper helps will be seen.

Industry defenders argue that antibiotics in animal feed are good for the public: animals get bigger faster, and that keeps prices of meat down.

Humans get bigger too. One telling piece of research took place in France. It was observed that many patients with a type of heart disease called infective endocarditis who were put on a popular antibiotic gained significant weight in the weeks and months afterward.[5] Earlier studies showed similar growth effects in children with the long-term use of antibiotics, most notably the popular tetracycline, in results that were noticed as far back as the 1950s.[6]

Those are examples of how antibiotics can directly cause weight gain. But many medications cause weight gain, as was seen in an earlier chapter. The question is whether the trickle-down effect can cause harm.

In other words, does a hamburger or glass of milk contain antibiotics? Or their residues? Can we be exposed to antibiotics—and their fattening qualities—by eating meat or drinking milk from an animal that has been on long-term antibiotics?

The answer is uncertain.

For example, one study in the Netherlands showed that pigs had "residues of tetracycline," which can cause allergic reactions and microflora upset in people eating its meat. However, authorities believe salmonella or other toxins in pork are more threatening than reactions or even energy disturbances from antibiotics.[7]

Drug residues are monitored in the United States by the FDA. Violations occur when the animal—usually a dairy cow—is killed for meat before the drug works its way out of the body. Two questions arise: at what level do drug residues disrupt metabolic rhythms to the point of gaining weight? Which antibiotics are most likely to cause weight gain? While these are not easily answered, low doses are turning out to be just as harmful as big ones, an unwelcome discovery that is upending the toxicology field. However big or small the effect, these antibiotic growth promoters in animals may end up in our food. Eating meat and drinking milk delivers them to us. And we may be gaining just like our animals.

GROWTH HORMONES

If you missed the documentary *Food, Inc.*, you may think that the quaint Klein farm that I visited is typical. Think again. Most modern farms, as the film depicts, are industrial operations that use precision agricultural and engineering systems to achieve higher crop harvests and heavier meat and milk yields. Their methods make for delicious food that is inexpensive and safe from deadly pathogens.

But new breeding techniques and overcrowded pens can be a living hell for the animals. Witness: chickens too large-breasted to walk, cows standing knee-deep in manure, and fish in tanks so packed a hook would be merciful.

And humans pay a price too. There is growing suspicion that methods that put weight on animals do the same for humans eating them.

We already saw how antibiotics increase weight in animals.

Growth hormones are another way to put on weight quickly. Hormones are given to cattle for two reasons: more meat and more milk. American farmers have been using synthetic growth hormones since 1994 and natural ones much longer, a practice that rewards with foods both plentiful and affordable. A pound of sirloin beef can be cheaper than a pound of tomatoes in a US supermarket. This alone presents an obesity link in that people eat more calorie-dense meat when they can afford it.

Yet the controversy about hormone use in agriculture extends beyond economics. The FDA asserts that the hormones are well tested and safe. Opposition groups argue that hormones pose several health risks, ranging from early puberty to cancer, and, more recently, obesity.

First, take a look at what's going in the dairy world. Cows naturally produce a hormone called bovine somatotropin (BST). In 1993, agricultural giant Monsanto used recombinant DNA technology to make a synthetic version named rBST. When the artificial hormone is added to feed, cows produce 10 to 15 percent more milk.[8] The higher volumes are a boon for poor countries but a dubious achievement for a rich place like the United States, where the government buys up surplus milk to support prices. Still, all that extra milk for a dose of rBST is not a bad return for the dairy farmer.

But it's not so great for the animals. Cows tend to get inflamed udders, a condition called mastitis, when given hormones and as a result require antibiotics. They have other problems too. A large-scale study from the Canadian Veterinary Medical Association found not only a 25 percent increase in mastitis but also a 40 percent drop in fertility and a 55 percent rise in risk for lameness.[9] Based on the health and welfare of animals, their use is banned in Canada, Japan, the European Union, Australia, and New Zealand.

Monsanto's evolution from chemical mastermind of two highly toxic substances—polychlorinated biphenyls (PCBs) and dioxin (Agent Orange by-product)— to biotechnologist altering the world's food supply was extensively reported by Pulitzer winners Donald Barlett and James Steele for *Vanity Fair* magazine in 2008. In the article titled "Monsanto's Harvest of Fear," the duo wrote that "scientists are concerned by the lack of long-term studies to test the synthetic hormone's impact, especially on children. A Wisconsin geneticist, William von Meyer, observed that when rBGH was approved the longest study on which the FDA's approval was based covered only a 90-day laboratory test with small animals. 'But people drink milk for a lifetime,' he noted."[10]

Use of the recombinant supplement continues to be contentious. The Codex Alimentarius Commission, a United Nations body that sets international food standards, has refused to approve rBST as safe.

Still, rBST milk is considered safe by the World Health Organization, the American Medical Association, the American Diabetic Association, and regulatory agencies in 50 countries.[11]

Nevertheless, many giant retailers—including Starbucks, Publix, and Walmart—are going rBST-free in response to consumer concern. Monsanto is fighting back—unsuccessfully in some places—to have rBST-free advertising removed from milk cartons.[12]

Whereas level of butterfat in the milk from rBST-treated cows is just slightly higher, the basic nutrient content of milk doesn't appear to vary much.[13] Growth hormone may not change the big nutrient picture but it works behind the scenes in sneaky ways. First, rBST nudges production of insulin-like growth factor 1 (IGF-1). This speck of a hormone is different than its namesake, insulin, which plays with sugar. IGF-1 promotes growth in almost every cell in the body. This may be quite nice if brain cells are affected but not so good if cancer cells are.

The IGF-1 in cow's milk is absorbed by humans.[14] In a 2010 review paper, cancer researchers at the Medical University of South Carolina wrote that "dysregulation of the IGF system is well recognized as a key contributor to the progression of multiple cancers."[15]

Because of its cheerleading role in growth, IGF-1 in milk is suspected in the obesity epidemic. Researcher Bodo Melnik at the Department of Dermatology, Environmental Medicine and Health Theory at the University of Osnabrück in Germany contends that milk protein consumption causes excessive insulin release after meals and leads to permanently increased IGF-1 serum levels. "Insulin/IGF-1 signalling," he writes, " is involved in the regulation of fetal growth, T-cell maturation in the thymus, linear growth, pathogenesis of acne, atherosclerosis, diabetes mellitus, obesity, cancer and neurodegenerative diseases, thus affecting most chronic diseases of Western societies."[16]

Others think differently. Terry Etherton, head of the department of Dairy and Animal Science at Pennsylvania State University, told Richard Laliberte, who wrote in *Weight Watchers* magazine:

"What's interesting about IGF-1 is that your own body is making it right now, and it's the exact same kind in milk. You would have to drink 100 quarts of milk a day to equal the amount of IGF-1 in your saliva."[17]

A 2008 study published in the *Journal of the American Dietetic Association* and sponsored by the Monsanto Company sampled store-bought milk across the United States and reported that organic, rBST-free, and conventional milks were not much different. Organic milk had less IGF-1 than either rBST-free milk or conventional milk: 2.73 versus 3.04 versus 3.12 all in nanogram per milliliter (ng/mL), respectively.[18]

Somewhat similar, not a huge difference, but over a lifetime? That's one more unanswered question in the synthetic hormone controversy.

Growth Hormones in Your Meat

In addition to increasing milk, hormones can make beef cattle grow faster and make meat leaner. The FDA reports, "Since the 1950s, the [FDA] has approved a number of steroid hormones for use in beef cattle and sheep." Some are identical to the hormones already in your body: estrogen, progesterone, and testosterone. Others are synthetic including zeranol and trenbolone acetate. Inserted as pellets on the animal's ear, the drugs are then discarded at slaughter. "No steroid hormones are approved for growth purposes in dairy cattle, veal calves, pigs, or poultry."[19]

Much of the outcry from the public has been because of the possible effects on children, especially in the realm of sexual development and reproduction. Children may be more sensitive to toxins because of their greater surface area per pound, higher metabolic rates, and maturing bodies.

The fears arose more than three decades ago, in a country where little girls wear ankle socks and carry dolls for much of their childhood. In 1977, girls in a northern Italian city were growing breasts and pubic hair at an early age. Town officials, spurred on by alarmed parents, asked whether the veal and poultry in school lunches may be the cause. Investigations led to no scientific conclusions, but when veal-based baby food turned up with residues of illegal synthetic hormones in 1980, the furor forced boycotts and bans.[20]

By the nineties, in the aftermath of the mad cow scare, the European Union banned the import of all beef that contained artificial hormones. Yet across the water, the FDA insisted that animals given growth hormone posed no danger. The FDA stands behind toxicology tests with established safe levels of hormone residues and regulations to enforce those marks.

Laliberte reported the following in the *Weight Watchers* magazine article: "'Residues in meat are really, really small—at the picogram level,' Etherton adds . . . 'There's no evidence of increased risk to the consumer or any human health effects at those levels,' he says."[21]

Nanogram or picogram: Either one is tiny. But whether either is small enough not to monkey with our bodies is the big question. A cadre of concerned scientists say low doses can be just as harmful. In a 2012 analysis headed by Laura Vandenberg at Tufts University, doses of estrogen disrupting chemicals not usually even tested were linked to a wide range of diseases including obesity.[22]

"There truly are no safe doses for chemicals that act like

hormones, because the endocrine system is designed to act at very low levels," Vandenberg told *Environmental Health News.*[23]

Thus, chemicals can be destructive in minute amounts even when benign at high amounts. Their role in obesity may add up.

Antibiotic residues and growth hormones sound threatening. Eating food exposed to them doesn't seem like a good idea. But other additives hiding in plain view may also best be avoided because they are potentially harmful or just less than benign. Plenty of them.

Additives used by food processors make a very long list: acidulants, antimicrobials, anticaking agents, buffers, chelating agents, clarifying agents, coloring agents, emulsifiers, enzymes, fillers, flavoring agents, flavor enhancers, gases, leavening agents, nutritive and nonnutritive sweeteners, propellants, preservatives, salts, and sequestrants, stabilizers, thickeners, texturizers, and tracers. One estimate places the tally over 2,000 strong. There are excellent reasons to use most of these: Better taste, longer shelf life, and defense against pathogens are the major ones.

Undeniably, food additives can also be helpful.

In 1958, the FDA established a list of 700 risk-free substances that were exempt from testing. This list is called GRAS (Generally Regarded As Safe). Unfortunately some thought to be harmful remain on the list.[24]

HIGH-FRUCTOSE CORN SYRUP

In 1983, the FDA awarded high-fructose corn syrup the coveted GRAS status for use in food and reaffirmed that ruling in 1996. Nevertheless, the HFCS story has proven to be less than sweet.

Forty years ago farmers across America were up to their ears in corn. Uncle Sam (really Earl Butz, the secretary of agriculture at the time) had deregulated export and trade of grains. Out came the hay and in went more profitable corn and soybeans. Farmers fed corn to cows. Animals for which grazing on grasses was long written in their dining history were now fed starchy corn in the confined mosh pits of industrial warehouses. Another big idea came from the lab: all this corn could be used as a sweetener if its chemical structure could be tweaked. The resulting high-fructose corn syrup seemed like a gift from the geek gods: it was cheaper than sugar, enhanced texture, tasted good, and lasted longer on the supermarket shelves.

Consumption of HFCS soared in the United States. According to USDA figures, HFCS has replaced 50 percent of all the traditional table sugar sucrose since 1970.

HFCS poured into soft drinks, sports drinks, fruit punches, pastries, and countless processed foods. In some cases it was added to foods not generally known to be sweet such as crackers and condiments. And possible the biggest beneficiaries of HFCS, soda and other sugary beverage companies, saw sales explode due to their lower cost.

As a result, total sugar, including sucrose and HFCS, increased by about 15 percent over the past four decades in the United States.[25]

The International Sugar Organization reports that the world average per capita sugar consumption has increased by a similar 16 percent over the past 20 years. Asian countries consumed 50 percent more sugar in that time but total per capita is still higher in South America, Oceania, and Europe.[26] Africa, traditionally low on the sweet-tooth scale, is acquiring one as sugary sodas flood the continent.

While this calorie increase from more sugar explains some of the rise in obesity, HFCS itself is also under scrutiny.

What is HFCS?

HFCS starts out as cornstarch. Companies use enzymes or acids to break down the starch into its glucose subunits. Then other enzymes convert some glucose to fructose.

HFCS is about half fructose and half glucose—exactly the same as ordinary table sugar called sucrose. So far, no reason to push all the blame on the new guy.

Indeed, we have other big sources of fructose in our diets such as fruit and honey. Fructose has the same chemical formula as glucose—the molecule in our blood ($C_6H_{12}O_6$)—but because of a slight chemical variation, it is used differently by the body: it heads right to the liver, where it becomes glucose, glycogen, lactate, and fat.

FRUCTOSE AND METABOLISM

Fructose may be to blame. How could this be? Isn't fructose the sugar we find in fruit? How could the sweetness in an apple or banana be making us fat?

The concern stems from two areas:

1. More fructose.

There is much more fructose in the food supply these days, coming from the addition of high-fructose corn syrup in many foods—even in a cracker, which isn't sweet—and increased consumption of sugary foods. See, fructose makes things taste better, so we eat more. Food producers know this, so they add fructose to processed foods that aren't even in the sweet club.

2. Metabolic changes

In mice and rats, a high-fructose diet leads to the development of obesity, diabetes, and dyslipidemia.

In humans, when consumed as part of a high-calorie diet, fructose can raise triglycerides in the blood, cause insulin resistance, and increase fat both in the liver and hips. Fructose, unlike table sugar or sucrose, is shunted straight to the liver. This little joy ride doesn't end well: the liver makes more fat and sends it back out into the blood where insulin resists the added work. Result: obesity.

For fruit lovers, this is not good news. But wait: fructose in fruit is not the same as the fructose flowing from corn syrup. The body sees them differently. Just as it confuses our cells, it is also difficult for scientists to parse; free fructose in HFCS is different than bound fructose in fruits or table sugar. Free fructose may be trouble.

Take a look at some of the newer research on fructose:

Fructose may not satisfy our appetites. Fructose is not glucose. It deals with key hormones differently. These three hormones are insulin, leptin, and ghrelin—all central to feeling satisfied after a meal or snack.

First, insulin response is lower—fructose carries a much lighter glycemic load than glucose—and this will impact satiety.

Second, leptin, the hormone that subdues appetite, responds

differently to fructose. Meals with fructose elicit less leptin than meals containing the same amount of glucose.[27]

High fructose intake not only triggered less leptin, the leptin it did evoke was not doing its usual job, an inertia called leptin resistance. How do we know this? Rats given leptin shots didn't lose their appetites when fed a fructose-rich diet. They were leptin resistant.[28]

Third, fructose impacts ghrelin—the only hormone known to increase appetite. Fructose-containing meals were less able to quash ghrelin than meals containing the same amount of glucose.[29] This could mean a bigger appetite with high-fructose diets.

And here's another piece of the puzzle: glucose is the primary fuel for the brain. Levels of glucose may be the litmus test telling the brain about the metabolic and nutritional state of the organism. Glucose tamps down food intake. But when fructose was infused into mice instead of glucose, the opposite happened—increased food intake.[30]

A 2013 study from the Yale University School of Medicine used MRIs to look at appetite centers of the brain after glucose or fructose ingestion in 20 adult volunteers. There were distinct differences in blood flow, insulin, and other appetite markers.[31]

Fructose may also change the speed of our inner engines. Mice on fructose water gain more fat than do mice given the same calories as sucrose.[32]

Ten weeks of fructose-sweetened beverages led to reduced resting energy expenditure in overweight men and women in another study.[33]

Also, fructose raises uric acid concentrations in humans and rodents. One unique aspect of fructose is that it is the only sugar that raises uric acid concentrations.[34] Uric acid will be familiar to you if you ever had a bout with gout, a painful form of arthritis in the joints. Inflammation may be the link to the obesity discussion.

For a more detailed look at a role for fructose in worldwide obesity, read an excellent 2010 review article from researchers at the University of Lausanne in Switzerland titled "Metabolic Effects of Fructose and the Worldwide Increase in Obesity."[35]

HFCS is thirty years new to the food supply; in that time,

obesity rates have soared. It could be the excess calories or it could be the way the HFCS is metabolized. Or could it be corn?

Crunching reams of data, researchers found a correlation with the entry of bioengineered corn into the food chain and obesity epidemic.[36] Repercussions may come with genetically modified foods (GM foods), which have been spliced and diced to resist disease and to add value. Whereas most European countries reject these foods, the United States had embraced the practice, most notably but not limited to corn and soybeans. In fact, most processed foods contain plants that have been genetically modified. Pick up a box of cereal, cookies, or salad dressing and read the label: no sign of its genetic manipulation, but it is there. Labeling requirement measures proposed in California were defeated in November of 2012 after negative advertisements from food and technology companies bombarded the voters. According to the *New York Times* online: "With so much at stake, food and biotechnology companies amassed $46 million to defeat the measure, according to MapLight, an organization that tracks campaign contributions. Monsanto, the largest supplier of genetically engineered seeds, contributed $8.1 million. Kraft Foods, PepsiCo and Coca-Cola each contributed at least $1.7 million."[37]

Bioengineered crops are not going away.

On the basis of both per capita disappearance data and individual food records analyses, there is no doubt that fructose consumption has increased over the past four decades in the United States, that teenagers and young adults are the highest consumers, and that the sweetened beverages are the main dietary source of fructose.

Greg Critser wrote in his book *Fat Land*: "In what would prove to be one of the single most important changes to the nation's food supply, both Coke and Pepsi switched from a fifty-fifty blend of sugar and corn syrup to 100 percent high fructose corn syrup. The move saved both companies 20 percent in sweetener costs, allowing them to boost portion sizes and still make substantial profits."[38]

Not only was soda different, it was cheaper. A 32-ounce cup at 7-Eleven cost the same price as a 12-ounce cup. It's an incredible bargain not offered anywhere else on the planet but America; very few could refuse such an offer. So up, up, up went sugary beverage consumption, a line on a graph mirrored by obesity.

There are studies linking body weight and soft drink consumption. One big analysis of 88 published studies from Yale University showed a significant link.[39] But others don't. At least twelve studies showed no such relationship.[40] Coincidentally, those funded by the food industry showed less impact from sugary drinks.

All the while that corn was transforming cows, chips, and colas (not to mention coffers), soybeans were too. The bountiful new crops convinced poultry and fish farmers to feed their charges soybean meal. Soybeans were pounded into soy flour to make breads and processed baked goods. Soy proteins joined hamburgers and chicken patties. Hydrolyzed vegetable proteins were stirred into sauces and soups, and soybean oil streamed into products in restaurants and on supermarket shelves.

It doesn't sound so bad—had we not learned from the lean and long-lived Japanese that soy is good? It is, up to a point, say experts, just like corn. Soy in the diet can lower cholesterol levels, but when radical changes happen quickly to our food supply and our diets, the outcomes are uncertain. Soy contains two naturally occurring chemicals, genistein and daidzein, two phytoestrogens that can inhibit the formation of fat cells. However, a 2013 finding from Denmark found that mice fed salmon raised on soybean oil showed insulin resistance and more fat accumulation in the liver.[41]

Also there is evidence that soy can feed tumors making the level in the food supply a concern.[42]

Tofu, miso, and tempeh: if these mess with the metabolism, the vegetarian world will reel in disappointment. But as with many nutrients, it just may be that eating whole soy foods naturally—rather than soy powders packed into smoothies or sports bars—may be the answer.

FATS

Quick review: Fat has an obvious role in obesity. Gram for gram, it supplies nine calories to only four for either carbohydrate or protein. It's packed with energy. Calorie-wise, the fat in a potato chip is no different than that in your imported olive oil. But slight twists in chemistry make the chip bad for your heart and the olive oil beneficial.

Fats and oils have been studied extensively, mostly in connection to heart disease. Whether from a plant or animal source, each fat starts with a carbon chain. Whether or not hydrogen atoms fill up or "saturate" those chains specifies a path in the body. Many saturated fats lead to clogged arteries, high cholesterol, and heart disease. As do trans fats. Monounsaturates, the Mediterranean menu stars, are heart healthy. Polyunsaturates break into different categories including omega-3 and omega-6 and are generally helpful depending on the ratio. Different fats and oils mean different things for the body. As a rule with many exceptions, liquid fats including olive and peanut oil are healthier than solids including butter and ghee.

The structure of dietary fatty acids, chain length, degree of unsaturation, position, and configuration of the double bonds seem to affect metabolism.

You are not alone if you find it all very confusing. Fatty acids and all their hijinks are fresh faces in science. Teasing out their true personalities may take some time.

Could the changes in quality of dietary fat in our food supply today, and not just the quantity, be related to the risk of obesity?

Researchers at the University of Montreal asked that exact question, publishing their results in the journal *Obesity* in 2008.

After combing through many reports they came up with this: some fatty acids are used, while others are more likely to be stored, even when comparing diets containing equal calories.

The authors concluded: "The rising biological plausibility linking dietary fat quality and risk of obesity, together with the rather recent addition of fatty acids content in food composition tables, support the need for major epidemiological studies in that area."[43]

Thus, while all fatty acids add an equal number of calories, they affect metabolic systems quite differently.

Our central question remains: is anything different about dietary fat today that could account for or contribute to the precipitous rise in obesity over the last three decades?

To be sure, many new fats have flooded our food supply.

The first offenders are the trans fats, a so-called "frankenfood" because of its lab origins and frightening results. Virtually nonexistent a century ago, trans fats slipped into margarines, fast food fries, cookies, commercial pastries, and countless other processed foods. Labeling laws wrestled from the FDA by a decade of pressure from Michael F. Jacobson and his nonprofit Center for Science in the Public Interest revealed hundreds of hiding places.[44] Trans fats raise bad LDL cholesterol and lower the good HDL. Their clear connection to heart disease spurred activists to call for reform. In addition, the huge tide of trans fats into the world's food supply may have no small connection to the rise in obesity. Research shows a connection in monkeys—more abdominal fat and insulin resistance—but further study may fade as the damage may be done.[45]

Once the darlings of the processed food world, trans fats have been cast out of many corporate kitchens. Local and state governments have weighed in, many banning them outright. McDonald's took the trans fats out of their frying oil; other fast food conglomerates and restaurants followed. Of course, they remain in many products, hiding as hydrogenated oils. In developing countries, people are often too busy getting enough to eat to care about the double bonds in their cooking oil.

Another change is the amount of omega-6 polyunsaturated fats in our diets. It dwarfs omega-3s—ones found in fish—now that food animals have switched from grazing on grasses and seeds to eating grains.

A brief mention of a fat substitute in our food supply: Proctor and Gamble promised much when they advertised fat-free potato chips containing the additive olestra. Unfortunately, this compound which travels undigested through the gastrointestinal tract, delivered hard-to-ignore malabsorption. This malabsorption led to the loss of needed vitamins and phytochemicals as well as perfectly good underwear. Whether or not this converted sugar molecule has messed with our metabolisms is under investigation. It could be that fooling the taste buds may not be such a good idea as is seen in artificial sweeteners. The body craves more.

Whether or not these changes are adding pounds will be determined. Meanwhile, it is prudent to remember that no matter how much we hear that olive oil is good and lard is bad, it is best to use small amounts whatever you choose.

MONOSODIUM GLUTAMATE

In my house, a meal of Chinese takeout meant you may be back in the kitchen in a few hours, scavenging for leftovers. Something about it made you hungry again. I figured it was the heaping portions of bamboo shoots and bean sprouts, fibrous no-calorie fillers, but a closer look showed equally big helpings of the fatty stuff: an order of kung pao chicken can top 2,000 calories and a day's worth of fat grams. No, some other ingredient in Chinese takeout was making us hungry.

Monosodium glutamate (MSG), a simple food additive better known for sparking allergic reactions or Chinese Restaurant Syndrome, may be the cause.

First, what is MSG and why is there so much in our food?

MSG is a form of a simple amino acid that is a building block of protein.

In 1908, Japanese chemist Kikunae Ikeda found that an amino acid called glutamic acid was giving the flavor to the seaweed "konbu," a soup essential that had been used for many centuries in Japan.

Since then the sodium salt of glutamic acid, or MSG, has been used as a seasoning around the world. Worldwide MSG consumption has increased dramatically in recent decades.[46] It's no surprise because MSG makes food taste better. It does this by tricking your tongue using a little-known fifth basic taste: umami.

Many amino acids are tapped to add flavor and intensity to foods and condiments. Artificial sweetener aspartame is S-aspartic acid, and S-phenylalanine. Soy sauce is essentially hydrolyzed soy or wheat protein, and "hydrolyzed vegetable protein" is widely used as a flavor component of many snack foods. Barbecue potato chips can contain cottonseed oil, sugar, dextrose, soy flour, salt, monosodium glutamate, paprika, onion powder, hydrolyzed soy protein, calcium silicate, partially hydrogenated soybean oil, caramel color, natural flavoring, natural hickory smoke flavor, garlic powder, calcium silicate, salt, sulfites, and, yes, potatoes, which actually are the first and heaviest ingredient.[47]

The glutamate in MSG is slightly different than the glutamate naturally coupled with other amino acids in foods. The versions are handled differently by the body. Also, glutamate in MSG is quickly absorbed whereas in food it has to go through the slow churn of digestion.

MSG has been linked to obesity in animals for several decades. Now research is a step closer in showing a connection in humans.

Animal Research

MSG-treated mice ate almost twice as much as controls. The marked interference with appetite could be a link to the obesity epidemic.[48]

Human Research

While the FDA rejects any dangers, MSG has been linked to weight gain in humans. In a 2008 study, 752 healthy middle-aged men and women were randomly selected in three rural villages in China. Most prepared their foods at home without use of commercially processed foods. Interviewers weighed MSG amounts added in food preparation. Diet, exercise, smoking and other variables controlled for, overweight was significantly higher in MSG users than non-users.

Dr. Ka He of the University of North Carolina who conducted the research said the results showed an association but not a cause-effect relationship.[49]

In a 2011 survey, also by He and colleagues, of more than 10,000 adults in China observed for more than five years, those who ate the most MSG (about five grams a day) were 30 percent more likely to become overweight in that time.[50]

Just as most other suspects in this book, MSG may have the power to change normal rhythms of appetite and energy metabolism. Even if subtle—which often means undetected—these changes can add up to weight gain.

Here's how MSG funds its pounds of flesh:

- Foods taste better with MSG, so we eat more.

- Leptin, that CEO of appetite, falls asleep on the job. It is thought that chronic MSG intake swamps neurons and disrupts the hypothalamic signaling cascade of leptin action, causing leptin resistance. Leptin's role is to alert the brain to stop eating. Leptin resistance is like a teenager with an iPod: she just doesn't hear you. Your body doesn't "hear" leptin telling it to stop eating, so you go on eating.

- Insulin is disrupted by MSG. Animal studies have shown that dietary MSG causes insulin resistance.

But wait, there's more to this MSG-obesity connection.

This next finding is disturbing. What if your mother's fondness for moo shu pork while pregnant can portend a less than lean adulthood for you? German researchers suggest that damage from MSG may take place before birth, setting the individual up for a lifetime of fighting a thrifty gene bent on adding weight.[51]

You may wonder this: if MSG is so fattening, why have Asian people typically been lean? Scientists involved in the China studies above asked the same thing. They suspect that the hypocaloric nature of their foods and increased exercise blunts the effect. Nevertheless, as incomes and calorie counts rise, obesity rates are surging as well, especially in China.

Abstaining from Chinese takeout isn't the answer. MSG lurks in hundreds of processed foods including bouillon cubes, packaged soups, and salty snacks. The last section of this chapter will show how to hunt for MSG and all its guises on food labels. Although evaluations conducted by the FDA and the World Health Organization concluded that MSG was a safe food ingredient for the general population, others are doubting its place in a healthy diet.

OTHER FOOD ADDITIVES

There may be other food additives upsetting our finely tuned system of appetite and metabolism.

One area that has been amply researched, mainly focused on links to cancer, is nonnutritive and low-nutrient sweeteners. These include saccharin, aspartame, and sucralose, the last new in 1999. You may know them by their brand names of Sweet'N Low, Equal, and Splenda.

More than 6,000 new products with noncaloric artificial sweeteners were launched in the United States between 1999 and 2004.[52] By 2013, sucralose was an ingredient in more than 3,500 products according to the online database at Foodfacts.com.[53]

The rise in obesity parallels the widespread use of these artificial sweeteners, an irony not missed in the soda aisles.

All are meant to supply sweetness without the calories. Fair enough. If a diet soda takes the place of regular one, calories are cut out of the diet, correct? Not necessarily, some say.

While people often choose these products to lose weight, artificial sweeteners may do the opposite. In 2010, Qing Yang at Yale University looked at studies behind the claim. In a first sign of trouble, the reviewer found that several large-scale studies showed weight gain with artificial sweetener use.[54]

One reason may be this: feeling virtuous with a diet food or beverage, the dieters reward themselves with extra calories in other foods. This was observed in a controlled setting; knowingly ingesting aspartame was associated with increased overall energy intake, suggesting overcompensation for the expected caloric reduction.[55]

Another problem was suspected: Natural and artificial sweeteners activate both reward pathways and taste receptors in different ways. Yang writes:

> Sweetness decoupled from caloric content offers partial, but not complete, activation of the food reward pathways. Activation of the hedonic component may contribute to increased appetite. Animals seek food to satisfy the inherent craving for sweetness, even in the absence of energy need. Lack of complete satisfaction, likely because of the failure to activate the postingestive component, further fuels the food seeking behavior.[56]

Thus these fake sugars with no calories do nothing for the satiety centers. A million years of evolution will not be easily fooled. Meanwhile, the nonnutritive sweetener keeps the taste buds on high alert for more sweet flavors, perhaps candy or cake next time. Because we prefer flavors we repeatedly taste, artificial sweeteners may lead to sugar craving and sugar dependence.

Artificial sweeteners have left a bitter aftertaste. Not only have they failed to help us lose weight, these imposters may be making us gain.

PACKAGING

Thus far in the chapter, we have looked at how chemicals linked to obesity enter our systems through the food supply: raising livestock or growing crops; improving flavor, color, texture, and other sensory pleasures of our groceries; prolonging shelf life; and reducing costs.

Another colossal change to our food entourage in the last 30 years is in packaging. Processing has ushered in plastic and other fossil fuel-based synthetics that lead to changes in our bodies, one of which may be obesity.

The damage of "progress" is stark in Egypt, where I live. In the rural villages that dot this arid land, women buy chicken wrapped in paper, toss vegetables in a cotton sack, and come dinnertime, serve rice in a clay pot and pour water from a ceramic pitcher. Contrast this to big-city Cairo, where in supermarkets meat and vegetables are sold on Styrofoam plates, sodas come in plastic and cans, and most everything else is entombed in cheap plastic wrap. Much of this detritus ends up in landfills, seas, or in the streets—waste disposal posing a daunting challenge in a desert country new to such heaps of garbage.

Even worse, the ecological madness doesn't end with a trashed landscape. Modern packaging is leaking harmful chemicals into our food.

One is phthalate, a chemical used to soften plastics. Each year, many billion pounds of phthalate esters are created and find their way into our cells through food and the way it's processed, packaged, stored, or heated.

Scientists here found that traditional hot Egyptian food such as *koushary* and *ful medams* served in plastic bags contained detectable levels of harmful phthalates.[57]

Phthalates can also be found in perfumes, hairsprays, insect repellants, medical supplies, and children's toys, as well as many industrial applications. It can be ingested, inhaled, or absorbed through the skin.

It's no wonder that more than 75 percent of a US population sample had measurable levels of phthalate metabolite in their urine, suggesting wide exposure.[58] By 2008, the United States had banned six phthalates from use in toys including pacifiers, play bath items, soft books, dolls, and plastic figures.[59] One major concern with phthalates is their anti-androgenic effects. Recent research reported that young boys play behavior changed if they had been exposed to high levels of phthalates before birth. The study published in the *International Journal of Andrology* revealed that the boys were less likely to engage in play fighting and truck driving.[60] Whether this effect points to an end to war and monster truck rallies is not yet known.

The sheer ubiquity of these chemicals may contribute to obesity. Scientists found that the concentrations of several phthalate metabolites to be positively and significantly correlated to abdominal obesity in adult males in the United States.[61]

Another chemical group suspected of obesogenic traits is the parabens. Though primarily used in cosmetics, parabens may be found in a small number of foods: jelly coatings of meat, dried meat products, coatings for nuts, and liquid dietary supplements. According to FoodNavigator.com, their use may be limited due to price and sensory issues.[62]

Bisphenol A (BPA)

More than six billion pounds of BPA, found in polycarbonate plastics and epoxy resins, are produced every year; it leaches from food and drink packaging, baby bottles, cans, and bottle tops. Humans are widely exposed to BPA, and it appears to accumulate in the fetus. The CDC found BPA in the urine of over 95 percent of nearly 400 U.S. adults and children tested.[63]

As a plasticizer, BPA is not intentionally added to our foods, but it sure has ended up there. In humans it acts as an estrogen disruptor, messing with puberty, reproduction, and energy metabolism. It is a prime suspect in the world's obesity epidemic. Read the evidence in the third chapter.

SOLUTIONS

I must admit, this chapter depressed me. True, the plentiful food supply of the last few decades has fed many more people, but did it have to mean adding stuff that would make us obese? From antibiotic residues in my yogurt to pesticides on my strawberries to the bisphenol A in my water bottle, I felt under siege. Fear may prove to be the best diet yet.

Avoiding foods with suspect chemicals will help with weight loss, precisely because we may have nothing much left to eat or drink. But of course, we eat to live, and at times the opposite may be true, so education is key.

Read the excellent online site from nutrition watchdog Center for Science in the Public Interest. In a section called Chemical Cuisine, there is a long list of food additives and safety ratings along with a printable chart. Their popular *Nutrition Action Healthletter* will keep you apprised of the most important food safety and health issues.[64]

Learn what your government does to protect, police, or improve your food. Countries respond differently and not in the ways you would expect. The European Union was quick to act against broad antibiotic use in animals or synthetic growth hormones in their beef cattle. The United States with its more powerful business interests allows both. Bangladesh banned plastic bags; Japan loves them. Asians savor MSG; Canadians hate it.

Food conglomerates have rich lobbies, which strong-arm government regulators. For more on these fascinating and often despicable collusions, read New York University professor Marion Nestle's excellent book *Food Politics*.[65]

Buy organic. This simple rule will go a long way in jettisoning obesogens.

Meat and Dairy

The United States Department of Agriculture (USDA) requires meat, poultry, eggs, and dairy foods labeled "organic" to come from animals that have not received antibiotics or growth hormones.

Organic multi-ingredient foods: The USDA organic seal verifies that the product has 95 percent or more certified organic content. "If the label claims that it was made with specified organic ingredients, you can be confident that those specific ingredients are certified organic."[66]

Don't be fooled by the words "natural" or other wholesome sounding adjectives.

Many countries do not have such regulations in place, so it is impossible to know what went into your hamburger. Faced with this mystery as well as knowing that meat is high in saturated fat and cholesterol, it may be advisable to push the delete button on this menu item.

Also, read labels. Some may say "no added hormones" or "milk from rBST-free cows."

Fruits and Vegetables

Organic food is produced without most conventional pesticides, bioengineering, ionizing radiation, or fertilizers made with synthetic ingredients or sewage sludge. Organic fruits and vegetables are farmed with natural methods.

According to the Environmental Working Group, you can reduce your pesticide exposure substantially by choosing organic versions of the fruits and vegetables shown in its tests to contain the highest pesticide load. The group calls them the Dirty Dozen Plus: In order of pesticide load, they are apples, celery, sweet bell peppers, peaches, strawberries, imported nectarines, grapes, spinach, lettuce, cucumbers, blueberries, potatoes, plus green beans and two leafy greens, kale and collards.

Almost all of the apples tested—98 percent—were teeming with pesticides. Buy the organic versions.

There's a Clean Fifteen, too, those with the least pesticide residue: onions, sweet corn, pineapple, avocado, cabbage, sweet peas, asparagus, mangoes, eggplant, kiwi, cantaloupe, sweet potatoes, grapefruit, watermelon, and mushrooms. For the full list and a downloadable booklet, visit the Environmental Working Group website: www.ewr.org.[67]

Other ways to reduce exposure are to buy from local farms,

wash well under water, remove the peel, and discard outer leaves.

One complaint about organic food is the price. This is mostly because of the smaller plantings. But as organic foods grow in popularity, prices should fall. Demand is rising at a fast clip. According to an Organic Trade Association survey, sales of organic food in the US "have grown from $1 billion in 1990 to $26.7 billion in 2009."[68]

Read Food Labels

Try not to eat anything with a label. A bit counterintuitive to what I as a nutritionist have been spouting about reading labels all these years, but it is a step in avoiding harmful additives and obesogenic plastic packaging. This would mean drastic change: Bread in brown paper, milk in a bottle, lettuce in a reusable sack. Start small and see how it can grow; buy local, cook from scratch, plant a garden, and eat out less often.

When you do eat something with a label, know these essentials:

The longer the ingredient list, the potential for harm is usually greater.

The ingredients are ordered by weight: the first ingredient is the biggest by weight.

Know that there are many ways to say sugar: glycerol, inversol, lactose, sorbitol, dextrose, malt, mannitol, and nearly a hundred more hidden sugars in your food. Try to steer clear of high-fructose corn syrup. Consumption is finally declining after many years of climbing.[69]

There are nearly as many disguises for MSG. It is one of those obesogens that lurks in many parts of a recipe. These ingredients can contain MSG: soy sauce, bouillon cubes and powder, malt extract, carrageenan, powdered milk, and gelatin. The best way to avoid MSG is to avoid processed and restaurant foods altogether. As that may be impossible, be on the lookout for the following: glutamic acid, vegetable protein extract, hydrolyzed vegetable protein, hydrolyzed plant protein, sodium caseinate, calcium caseinate, yeast extract, and yeast food, or nutrient and autolyzed yeast.[70]

Lose the taste for sweet and salty. Over time appetite for these two will wane. Use natural colors and flavor. Green and white teas contain catechins, fruits such as blueberries have anthocyanins, red grapes and wine boast resveratrol, and spice like turmeric contain curcumin; all provide health benefits of various stripes including improving blood glucose and lipid profiles, reducing insulin resistance, and obesity. Plant foods are a trove of phytochemicals yet to be discovered.

Packaging

You buy organic, avoid processed foods and try to do everything right. But then you buy that lovely pesticide-free, organic broccoli wrapped in plastic. When it comes to packaging and storing, here are a few rules:

- Shop with reusable bags. Read the tragic results on reuseit.com[71]

- Avoid plastic-wrapped foods. Ask that grocery items be wrapped in paper or reusable containers of glass, ceramic or safe plastics.

- Pay attention to canned foods. Many are lined with BPA, an estrogen disruptor that several countries have banned. According to the Environmental Working Group, canned chicken soup, infant formula, and ravioli have BPA levels of the highest concern. The United States is resisting pressure from public health groups but large companies including soup giant Campbell's are removing BPA from cans voluntarily. And those paper receipts: handle as little as possible; they are swimming in BPA.

As for your sturdy reusable water bottle: After college students drank out of a polycarbonate bottle (usually stamped with a #7 on the bottom) for just one week, their BPA levels jumped by nearly 70 percent, according to a study from Harvard University.[72]

Numbers to memorize: #7 may include BPA and #3 may contain phthalates. Plastics with recycling codes #2, #4, and #5 are safer.

- Avoid drinking hot beverages from Styrofoam or coated paper cups.

- Reheat foods in pots and pans on the stove. Microwave foods in glass or ceramic. Don't laminate your leftovers with plastic wrap in the microwave. And then there's the practice of using plastic plates, utensils, and cups and washing them and reusing. Use the good dishes. No one wants them after you're gone.

Writing this takes me back to the very beginning of this story, when I hiked the rocky canyons at the edge of Cairo. I stepped over soda cans and plastic bags littering a wilderness that had been pristine for millions of years. And on the way home, I saw many women, young and old, who were too heavy to walk more than a few steps. We had come a long way, but not the right way. It's easy to see that what is good for our planet is also good for our health. So easy to see, harder to do. Yet it's not impossible to choose the road not taken, a healthier one.

10

. . . .

YOU SNOOZE, YOU LOSE
WEIGHT: SLEEP & OBESITY

Our rhythms are off when we get poor or little sleep. Our distressed hormones respond by telling us to eat more.

BABY'S UP TOO LATE, BABY IS TIRED; TEENS FALL-ing asleep in class, teens napping after school; boomer friends with sleeping pills, custom mattresses, white noise machines, sleep coaches, zzzzz. . . . Sleep used to be so simple.

People are sleeping less these days. And the sleep they do get is not the best. All this tossing and turning isn't burning calories; in fact, it can make us gain weight. As we shall see, both quantity and quality of sleep can lead to obesity.

But first, what exactly is sleep? Fascinating as it turns out. Did you know that most fish sleep like night watchmen, one-half of their brains at a time so to keep watch for predators? Or that dolphins don't sleep for the first month after birth? Factoids like these are as endless as the number of species on the planet. Bats sleep during the day like vampires while humans like to sleep at nighttime. Quick review: Light and dark are the most powerful forces controlling life on our planet. Rotation of the earth around the sun imparts light and dark cycles of 24 hours; humans call it one day. All life forms respond to this light show with internal rhythms called circadian; these beats lay out daily tracks for sleep-wake cycles as well as body temperature, hormone secretion, and many other biological exploits.

Conducting this cellular symphony is a master clock, a mere snippet of tissue in the front of the brain. It works from the suprachiasmatic nucleus, which has proven to be as fabulous as its name. With light as its ruler, the clock synchronizes messages via nerves and hormones and hears from melatonin, serotonin, ghrelin, motilin, gastrin, cholecystekin and others by way of countless little clocks in the gut and beyond. The complexity of the clock system inside us all is worthy of a Nobel Prize for the persons unraveling its mechanisms. Much is still a mystery. A 2012 review from the University of Fribourg in Switzerland (of course) concludes:

"The interplay between the central neural and peripheral tissue clocks is not fully understood and remains a major challenge in determining how neurological and metabolic homeostasis is achieved across the sleep-wake cycle. Disturbances in the communication between the plethora of body clocks can desynchronize the circadian system, which is believed to contribute to the development of diseases such as obesity and neuropsychiatric disorders."[1]

Indeed, weight gain as well as elevated levels of insulin and leptin followed when researchers at Rockefeller University in New York City disrupted circadian rhythms in mice.[2]

So what do humans do? We batter this gift of innate Swiss precision with night shifts, caffeine, 24-hour texting, late-night television and all-night raves. Basically, we disturb the talk between the clocks. And that sets us up for obesity.

In the following pages, we will look at how little sleep humans are getting, why, and how the body gets fat when it is deprived of sound sleep.

PEOPLE ARE SLEEPING LESS

Wealthy countries have the luxury of proper statistics on sleep. America, for instance, has organizations devoted to the study of sleep, which itself may imply a problem. Many studies as well as wide-scale polling by the National Sleep Foundation (NSF) suggest that Americans are chronically sleep-deprived.

In the early 1900s, sleep time averaged almost nine hours. That number fell to less than eight hours by the late 1960s.[3] By 2002, the median sleep duration had declined to seven hours.[4] A more recent poll by the NSF in 2008 showed a further drop: average six hours and forty minutes per weeknight.[5]

That was the average, but many were short sleepers, getting fewer than six hours of shut-eye.[6] Researchers looked at time diaries (considered more accurate than recall) from eight studies conducted in the United States from 1975 through 2006. Percentages of short sleepers rose from 7.6 percent in 1975 to 9.3 percent in 2006.[7] Other countries appear more restful than America. When researchers looked at self-reported sleep times in Finland over a similar period, they found an 18 minute decline in sleep duration and no increase in short sleepers.[8] Another study done across the decades, this time in Sweden, reported a 15-minute decline in sleep time for the women over a 36-year period. But, interestingly, sleep problems doubled.[9]

Sleep Disturbances on the Rise

The majority of Americans polled in one NSF survey had sleep problems such as waking up and not being able to go back to sleep or waking up feeling unrefreshed. Overall, they spent an average of 21 minutes falling asleep on weeknights. More than 60 percent were getting less sleep than they thought they needed on weeknights, a number they estimated to be on average 7 hours and 28 minutes.[10] Exploding sales in sleep medications, special mattresses, and memory-foam pillows further attest to a big problem.[11]

WHY CAN'T WE SLEEP?

The most obvious answer goes back to the nineteenth century with the discovery of electricity. Artificial light and all its plugged-in progenies swept in and have hampered our natural hominid rhythms ever since. But it was not until the 1960s and the furied rise of the technological revolution that the restful rejuvenation of sleep took a real dive. People are now too busy to sleep. The Internet makes everything immediate and available 24 hours a day. Professions that were nine to five in the 1980s now expect an on-call response from their employees, whether journalists or garage mechanics. Pressure mounts to reply to work requests, Facebook friends, tweets, and emails. Fewer people take vacation, and more people work at night. Sleep is somewhat of a competitive sport: too much sleeping is looked down upon as lazy, especially in America where sleep time has dropped drastically. High achievers report needing only five hours; all-nighters get the job down. There are distractions, duties, and yet one more thief of sleep: insomnia caused by a slew of stimulants and stresses. Sleep is hopelessly out of fashion.

Screens Are to Blame

Remember when a screen was a metal netting that kept out the pests of summertime? Our newest screens let everything in: a whole world of entertainment, education, information, conversation, transactions, shopping . . . How did it happen that we greet the morning at the computer and say good night the same way? In Cairo during the revolution, the government shut down the Internet for several days. The horror. There could be no idle watching of the overthrow on YouTube. No Facebook friends commiserating. No Twitter updates. That Mubarak miscalculation sent millions into Tahrir Square, adding momentum to the rebellion.

Point being, we need our screens. When the Internet goes down, we struggle. When electricity goes off—a common occurrence in the heat of Cairo—we downright panic. Especially in the evening. I've read by candlelight a few times, some Lincolnesque fun that lasts about five minutes. But mostly I wonder this: what on earth did people do before electricity? And then I go to sleep, because there is nothing else to do. And that is when the metaphorical lightbulb goes off: technology has changed us drastically in a short blip of biological history; its greatness has a dark side, part of which is poor health.

Television has been blamed for obesity for a long time now. But reaching back into history, we see that radio and before that, storytelling, were sedentary forms of entertainment as well. Why pick on television? Even as television replaces time that could be spent in active pursuits, researchers have found that actual couch time is not the only path to obesity.

What then? At least three changes in television culture qualify, all with timelines eerily similar to the obesity surge in the last three decades: Twenty-four-hour programming with hundreds of choices; cheap and abundant snack foods; and targeted marketing of junk and fast foods.[12]

The last may be the most fattening. Food is the most commonly advertised product on children's television. Kids see one food ad every five minutes during Saturday morning cartoons, according to one study.[13] And worse, almost all of these foods are of poor nutritional value.[14]

Marketers target children as young as two and it works. The typical first-grade child can already recognize and respond to more than 200 brands.[15] And much research shows that a child exposed to commercials is more likely to choose these foods.[16]

Thus watching a show such as *SpongeBob SquarePants* with commercials was linked to obesity, but watching videos or educational television without commercials was not, researchers found.[17] Obesity may be the result of commercials and not television.

Shutting off the television does lower weight. The interesting thing is that it is due to reduced calories rather than any jump in physical activity. Without constant cues to eat, the child eats less.[18]

Of course, the television screen has made way for a new kind of entertainment: the personal computer (PC). In widespread use for only about 20 years, a computer offers all sorts of fun attractions: streaming movies, socializing, gaming, and shopping. At one time these amusements involved an activity like walking to a theater, meeting friends at a park, bouncing a ball, or circling the racks at a department store. No more. It's much easier and usually more economical to do these things on a computer. And so each day we become more tethered to screens. In addition to fun, we are now required to tend to business and chores on the computer. Online banking and investing have unseated brick-and-mortar transactions. Insurance, travel, credit cards, taxes . . . almost everything can be done online.

Boys growing up in the last few decades have exceeded most reasonable limits in gaming. PlayStation and Xbox have claimed our young boys and their sleep like nothing else. Sure, it kept them off the streets and one study even claimed it made them better drivers with excellent response skills. But it made them sedentary and maybe even more tolerant of violence (first-person shooters). As for girls, they were fairly indifferent until MySpace and Facebook created the biggest online party a teen could ever want. Gaming and social media have exploded around the globe. More than a billion people use Facebook. All of this may be good for the global village but is it healthy for our personal collections of cells?

So far, the health implications are not good.

In addition to replacing physical exercise, gaming and social media sites expose users to advertisements for sweetened beverages and other unhealthy foods. Video game-playing strongly predicts weight status.[19]

Internet and computer use predicted overweight and obesity in an Australian study. After adjusting for many variables, including sedentary behaviors, participants who used the Internet and computer for three hours or more in the seven-day period tested were 1.5 times more likely to be overweight and 2.5 times more likely to be obese compared to nonusers.[20]

Screen time was also studied in Saudi Arabia, which has seen drastic changes in lifestyle in the last few decades. Modernization and great wealth have brought inactive hobbies and all the fast food that money can buy. Obesity rates are skyrocketing, as are diabetes and other chronic diseases.

Health authorities there looked at youths aged 14–19 in three cities in the Kingdom. The more screen time (television, video games, and computer) there was, the higher the consumption of fast foods, sugar-sweetened drinks, french fries and potato chips, cakes and donuts, candy and chocolate, and energy drinks. Females showed an especially strong correlation as well as a reduced intake of breakfast and vegetables, fruit, milk, and dairy products.

The researchers discovered that sedentary behaviors among Saudi adolescents were remarkably high. The American Academy of Pediatrics has issued guidelines recommending that screen time not exceed two hours per day. But 84 percent of males and more than 91 percent of females in this large sample of teenagers exceeded the two-hour daily screen time recommendation.[21] These numbers in Saudi Arabia are similar to the figures in Canada and the United States. Numbers no one is trying to emulate.

Screen time cuts into sleep time. This is one more way we gain weight. In 2011, the NSF conducted a study of newer technology and its impact on sleep.

The findings were troubling:

- 39 percent of Americans use their cell phones in their bedrooms before they go to sleep; people under 30 are most likely to do so.

- 10 percent say they get emails, texts, or calls interrupting sleep at least a few nights a week.

- Over 60 percent use laptops regularly within an hour of going to sleep, while more than one in three uses a computer in the bedroom. What are they doing? Skyping, surfing the Internet, watching movies, making spreadsheets, and checking Facebook.

How much sleep are they getting?

- Generation Z'ers (13–18): 61 percent say they get fewer than 8 hours nightly.

- Generation Y'ers (19–29) are more likely to get adequate sleep, yet 23 percent get fewer than the recommended 7 hours for this age group.

- Generation X'ers (30–45) and baby boomers (46–64) have similar sleep patterns: they get fewer than 7 hours on average.[22]

The result of all this poor sleep? Daytime sleepiness, napping, and caffeine use are all on the upswing.

If a mocha latte addiction was the only problem, there'd be no worries. But sleep deprivation leads to disease: hypertension, heart disease, diabetes, and cancer, as well as impaired performance and memory, impaired immune function, and increased risk of accidents.

And obesity. This is not some crazy theory. Without a doubt, short sleepers are heavier than those who sleep seven to eight hours. An imposing stack of reports from all over the world links changes in sleep to the obesity epidemic.[23]

Scientists Frank Hu and Sanjay Patel considered most of it in their chapter presented in Hu's excellent compendium titled *Obesity Epidemiology*.[24]

Take a look at a few of these studies:

Brazilian truck drivers: Truck driving is tough on the body. Sitting all day takes its toll as do long hours on the road. Of the 4,878 men surveyed, those who slept fewer than 8 hours a day were more likely to be obese.[25]

Iowan farmers: Of 990 workers surveyed, body mass index (BMI) was higher as sleep decreased.[26]

Japanese patients: In a small clinic sample, odds of obesity were nearly double for those sleeping fewer than 6 hours, the so-called short sleepers.[27]

French women: Of 1,469 women, short sleep duration was related to higher BMI.[28]

Spanish adults and adolescents: Of 1,772 people, those sleeping nine or more hours had a lower rate of obesity than did those sleeping six or fewer.[29]

United States: In a study of over 900 patients at clinics, a higher BMI was linked to fewer hours of sleep.[30]

Detroit, Michigan, sample: In this study of 3,100 people, researchers Singh and colleagues reported that those who slept six or fewer hours were at highest odds of being obese. And they noticed a curious thing: African-Americans slept less, much less than Caucasians; they were twice as likely to get no more than five hours sleep per night.[31] Another study, this time looking at 32,000 adults in the United States, also found a higher risk of sleep extremes in African-Americans.[32]

In the United States, certain minority populations have high rates of obesity. One in two African-American women, for example, is obese, higher than the general population.[33] Sleep habits may have something to do with these high rates.

Long-Term Evidence

Another way to get at the truth is to chart changes through time. This is called a longitudinal study. Several of these long-term studies link sleep debt and obesity.

One study followed 68,000 nurses in the United States over a 16-year period. A brief aside here on the powerful and voluminous data that have come from the Nurses' Health Study: My mother was a participant. She conscientiously filled out questionnaires for many years. She loved being a part of it and anxiously awaited the findings in academic journals. Nurses were chosen because they were known to be honest, intelligent, and reliable in sending the forms back (that's my mom). Science owes this group a big debt. On this subject, the data from the nurses showed that those reporting five and six hours of sleep a night gained more weight than did those with seven to nine hours.[34]

Another long-term, large-scale study is the National Health and Nutrition Examination Survey (NHANES I). Data from 18,000 adults aged 32–59 years revealed the least obesity with a moderate seven-hour snooze.[35]

A third longitudinal study followed 496 adults as they aged. Those with lower sleep times gained more weight over time.[36]

And in a Stanford study of more than 1,000 adults, for people sleeping fewer than eight hours, increased BMI was proportional to decreased sleep. The lowest BMI corresponding to about 7.7 hours of sleep per night.[37]

Scientists asked more questions: Could other medical conditions or medications contribute to the obesity? What effect does low income or high income have on the results? Do genes affect it? Age? Ethnicity?

Sleep and BMI were related regardless of these factors.

BIGGEST LOSERS

Children may suffer the most in this weary new world. They don't sleep enough. Even as their needs remain high and constant in crucial growing years, average sleep for young people has plummeted in recent decades. Why? Liberal parenting, heavy schedules, and a toy box full of electronic gadgets, which are more fun than a pillow.

How much sleep do kids need?

When given a chance, children between the ages of 10 and 17 will sleep for about nine hours. Younger children need more. But in recent surveys even the youngest children sleep fewer than nine hours.[38]

As sleep has dropped, childhood obesity rates have doubled and tripled in some places. Connection? Scientists think so.

French children: In 1,031 five-year-olds, shortened sleep duration was related to obesity.[39]

German children: Among 6,862 five- and six-year-olds, less sleep meant higher BMIs and body fat mass.[40]

Japanese schoolchildren: Of 8,274 children, shorter sleeps meant more weight.[41]

These studies controlled for parental obesity, television watching, and other fat builders.

Here's another way to study the sleep-obesity relationship:

United States children: 150 were followed from birth to age nine and a half. Those with shorter sleep times at age three and four were more likely to be overweight at the end of the study.[42]

Japanese children: 8,170 children were checked at three and then six years of age: short sleep duration, among other factors, meant more overweight kids.[43]

Texan adolescents: Of 383 young people aged 11–16 years, the obese adolescents had less sleep than the non-obese adolescents. For each hour of lost sleep, the odds of obesity increased by 80 percent.[44]

Not convinced yet?

Many more studies across five continents concur: for children, too little sleep can lead to obesity.[45]

Measuring sleep is no slacker's job. It can be surprisingly difficult getting an accurate read. Even if you isolate the sleepers and watch them sleep, a rather labor-intensive task, you can't be sure when they are sleeping or waking up or even pretending to sleep. A method called polysomnography can do that but is criticized because electrodes and recording devices may make sleep uncomfortable, thus shortening it. And then there is actigraphy, a device attached to a wrist or leg. It's less obtrusive, if you don't mind wearing a wristwatch or leg-shackle to bed. Most big studies rely on questionnaires to measure sleep.

Or they just join them at mealtime. That's right. Scientists can pick out sleep-deprived lab rats merely by observing how much they eat. The rats can't get enough: "hyperphagic" in science lingo. I myself am remarkably hyperphagic after a long red-eye flight, which is hard to explain given that I've just eaten three trays of fatty airplane food.

Sleep debt leads to all sorts of physical changes that favor weight gain. These changes can increase calorie intake, as in a post-flight feeding frenzy, or reduce energy output or even do both.

HOW DOES LACK OF SLEEP LEAD TO OBESITY?

Fatigue. How do you feel after waking before dawn with a newborn or staying up until four in the morning working on a school project? Tired, of course. And tired people aren't out training for marathons; they are listless couch lovers if they have that luxury. Though seemingly obvious, the fatigue that comes from little sleep has actually been studied in both children and adults. Sleepless nights lead to reduced physical activity.[46]

When healthy young men were restricted to four hours in bed for two nights, a decrease in daytime spontaneous physical activity followed.[47] But surprisingly, when physical activity is controlled, sleep debt is still linked to obesity per Nurses' Health Study data.[48] Being tired and lethargic alone is part of the problem but not the entire explanation.

Weight gain occurs over time and small changes in movement add up. But there are other changes.

Body temperature. Sleep loss causes a drop in core temperature: cold intolerance and shivering set in sooner in the sleep-deprived.[49] A recent experiment showed that the body will conserve energy when sleep-deprived. Healthy adults spent more than five weeks in a sleep lab at Brigham and Women's Hospital in Boston. After a period of normal sleep, they were allowed only 5.6 hours sleep per 24-hour cycle. The amount of energy the body used at rest, the resting metabolic rate, declined on average 8 percent.[50]

When adults were deprived of sleep in a 2013 collaborative experiment, total of all energy expenditure (includes resting and other activities) increased about 5 percent. Foraging for food was one popular activity for them as they ate more and gained an average of two pounds after just one week, in spite of more exertion. The good news: after they recovered sleep, weight slipped down as well as fat and carbohydrate intake.[51]

These men and women in the sleep lab showed other drastic changes during their time as lab rats. (Random hallway scurrying was not monitored).

Change in hormones. Sleep debt affects many hormones that may act on appetite, metabolic rate, and other systems of weight management. In addition to insulin, these include cortisol, growth hormone, thyroid-stimulating hormone, leptin, and ghrelin. Every one of them is distressed when we don't get our sleep.

Glucose and insulin. The people in the Boston sleep study showed increased insulin resistance after disturbed sleep: a 27-percent average drop in insulin secretion after eating, and then higher glucose levels.[52]

Other studies point to this faulty insulin response in the sleep-deprived. In one, men restricted to four hours of sleep for six nights had a 40-percent decrease in the rate of glucose clearance and a 30-percent reduction in insulin response.[53] Less severe restrictions of only a few hours short for two weeks had similar effects. Amazingly, healthy adults showed a diabetic profile just by sleeping too little. Deranged sugar and insulin can lead to weight gain.[54]

Why does sleep debt tamper with glucose and insulin? For one, sleep displays markedly different brain activity than an awake state. And this: the brain depends mostly on glucose for its energy, whereas other parts of the body can reach into fat and glycogen stores. During a fast, fully one-half of glucose use is by the brain. These levels are constant when asleep but plummet if you try to fast during the day—ask any Muslim during the month of Ramadan about brain fog. Nope, these precise sugar levels don't happen by magic.

The brain employs special methods to keep glucose steady while sleeping: glucose uptake, growth hormones, insulin sensitivity, and cortisol all fluctuate at different parts of the sleep cycle, making sure the brain is never deprived of its precious fuel.

During the first part (short wave sleep) of a proper sleep, there is a 30- to 40-percent drop in glucose uptake. That improves in the waking or rapid eye movement (REM) phase.

It is not surprising then that sleep loss will impact this sweet sonata. Cutting off the last half or delaying the start of sleep only confuses the players, as was seen in numerous studies.

Quality of sleep, not only quantity, matters when it comes to glucose control.

Cortisol, a stress hormone, courses through the body in a wave shape: high tide on awaking, ebbing throughout the day and then an abrupt surge near the end of the night. If you happen to wake in the middle of the night, there is a "pulse" in cortisol secretion. This 24-hour cycle is controlled by circadian clocks.

Shorter sleep duration was linked with disturbances in these hormonal and metabolic variables. Evening cortisol levels were highest when the subjects were in a state of sleep debt.[55]

Thyroid-stimulating hormone. During partial sleep deprivation, thyroid-stimulating hormone levels and the duration of its secretion have also been found to be blunted even when energy intake and activity levels were held constant.[56, 57]

Growth hormone. A pulse of growth hormone occurs at the beginning of sleep. This is slow-wave sleep. If sleep is disrupted, the growth hormone release is minimal or absent. This impact by sleep is most clear in men but is also detected in women.[58]

Two appetite hormones. Leptin is like a pair of tight pants; it tells us to stop eating. Because it reacts to meals, leptin is low in the morning and high at night. Secreted from fat cells, it increases energy burn and shrinks food intake. Leptin has its sleep-time levels like other hormones. Disruption of sleep will set off alarms in appetite control.

That is exactly what happened to rats after 15 days of sleep deprivation: leptin dropped and feeding rose.[59]

Humans showed leptin changes too. When subjects had only five hours of sleep, leptin levels were 15.5 percent lower than those sleeping eight hours.[60]

Likewise, in healthy young men at the University of Chicago restricted to four hours sleep, leptin levels were 18 percent lower than when they were allowed ten hours in bed.[61] Lower leptin means bigger appetite. The brain cries out for more fuel; hunger and appetite shot up more than 20 percent in these men. And more alarming was the bigger desire for energy-dense, high-carbohydrate foods.[62] Buckets of fried chicken and deep-fried Oreos never looked so good.

Ghrelin does the opposite of leptin: it signals you to eat. It's the hunger hormone. Ghrelin comes from the stomach; it drops after a meal and rises when another meal is needed. It also kicks up when sleep is short.

In the previous studies on leptin, researchers also checked ghrelin levels. This is what they found:

Ghrelin levels were almost 15 percent higher with five hours of sleep as opposed to eight hours.[63]

In the students limited to four hours for two nights, ghrelin levels increased by 28 percent in nine of the men. Lower leptin and higher ghrelin translate into bigger appetites. And remember, these men were seeking the most energy-dense foods.[64] Such foods are available all the time now: all night drive-thrus for everything from steak dinners to stacks of pancakes; 24-hour supermarkets with a smorgasbord of takeout from macaroni and cheese to pepperoni pizza; and of course, convenience stores for the incidentals of candy, soda, and chips. It's a problem when little sleep makes a big appetite.

Orexin is good at many things. It keeps us awake. It makes us eat. And it is tangled in the whole reward system that forms our desires. When orexin is deficient, humans and rodents have a hard time staying awake, a state called narcolepsy. This peptide shoots up when we are sleep deficient.[65] Orexin responds to leptin and glucose, linking it to energy systems. And then with its role in reward-related systems, orexin takes on even more importance.

Interestingly, a recent study in adolescents showed that poor sleep led to less reaction in the reward department, suggesting that the rewards were no longer exciting.[66] More stimuli were needed: More food, more treats, perhaps?

Researchers at Kanazawa University in Japan project that orexin system could be an important target for the management of obesity because it is "a critical regulator of sleep/wake states and of feeding behavior and reward processes."[67]

One more: *Obestatin* was discovered in 2005. It appears to do the opposite of ghrelin. It causes anorexia. It also regulates sleep as well as other duties.[68]

Albert Stunkard knows all about eating behavior. His name precedes the Center for Weight and Eating Disorders he founded at the University of Pennsylvania. The nonagenarian professor of psychiatry was the first to describe and develop treatments for binge eating disorder, which led to study of night eating syndrome, behaviors that intersect with short and disrupted sleep. More than 25 years ago, Stunkard and a colleague developed a questionnaire to measure dietary restraint, disinhibition, and hunger.[69]

Disinhibition is overeating in response to cognitive or emotional cues. Examples of disinhibition are eating half a chocolate cake when you break up with your boyfriend; going for thirds and fourths at the wedding buffet; or eating more to please your grandma.

French researchers adapted this survey to ask short-sleepers about their eating styles. They observed that having a high disinhibition eating behavior trait significantly increases the risk of overeating and gaining weight in those with short sleep duration.[70] This could explain why some short sleepers are rail thin—they have a different style. This concept is buttressed by more studies showing that sleep restriction increased snacking[71] and disinhibited short sleepers preferred sweet and high-fat foods.[72]

Consider this: the urge to snack on junk food may simply reflect short sleep clocks setting off alarms, which trigger stress responses and reward-seeking behaviors.[73]

Apparently overeating is not just a lack of self-control. Our rhythms are off when we get poor or little sleep. They are telling us to eat more.

Stunkard and a team at the University of Pennsylvania looked at night eating syndrome, which is overeating in the evening and then waking up at night and eating.[74] The women were kept in the lab for three nights. Food, glucose, and seven hormones (insulin, ghrelin, leptin, melatonin, cortisol, thyroid-stimulating hormone, and prolactin) were measured. The women lapsed into circadian cacophony with leptin and insulin showing delays of one to nearly three hours. But levels of ghrelin—the hormone that stimulates eating—were ahead of schedule by more than five hours. The authors surmise the changes "may result from dissociations between central (suprachiasmatic nucleus) timing mechanisms and putative oscillators elsewhere in the central nervous system or periphery, such as the stomach or liver."[75] In other words, the clocks are off. The big hand isn't talking to the little hand.

Such shifts in timing may also help explain eating changes when we are deprived of sleep quantity or quality.

But this being science, the chicken or the egg question is assured: instead of sleep debt causing obesity, could obesity be leading to short sleep?

In some cases, yes. Obesity is a risk factor for conditions that interrupt sleep including apnea, acid reflux, and congestive heart failure. Some obese people suffer from sleep apnea, a breathing disorder that cuts down on healthy sleep time. But many obese people don't have these disorders. Besides, the strongest connection for sleep debt and obesity is in children, who rarely have apnea.

SOLUTIONS

Solving this mess seems easy enough: get more sleep. Then we won't have metabolic and endocrine alterations including decreased glucose tolerance and insulin sensitivity, increased evening concentrations of cortisol, increased levels of ghrelin, decreased levels of leptin, increased hunger and appetite, and rampant obesity. Sleeping to lose weight is a marketer's dream. Who couldn't sell such a concept? NIH is tracking whether longer sleep of about seven and a half hours will figure in weight change for obese participants who averaged less than six hours a night when screened. The results will be interesting.[76]

Moreover, a good night's sleep will benefit all areas of your life. No more drowsy driving (which actually kills fewer than obesity) or accidents at the jobsite but smoother relationships, better school grades, and increased work performance. There is nothing much good about losing sleep.

For those with ample free time and ability to nod off when they hit the pillow, an earlier bedtime may be all it takes. But for the rest of the twenty-first century population who deal with texting in the middle of the night, Skype calls in the early morning, swing shifts and night shifts, or just too much to do, getting to bed for some sound sleep will take a plan.

- Establish a routine. The best sleepers don't deviate much.

- Switch off all electronics, including television, an hour before bedtime. Limit commercial television, especially for children, who are sponges for junk food marketing. Replace with any of the huge variety of wholesome DVDs available.

- Take a hot bath or shower right before bedtime.

- Exercise vigorously and every day if possible. But not too close to sleep time.

- Get checked for apnea and other things that go harrumph in the night.

- Darken the room. Follow the example of business hotels by adding blackout shades or drapes. Or wear the eye mask from the airplane.

- Turn on the quiet. *Money* magazine suggests that "if noise is a problem, skip the $200 white-noise machine and download TMSoft's White Noise app for your iPad or iPhone ($1.99, Apple). Just be sure to turn off the iPhone ringer or set it to 'airplane' mode." Or try earplugs.[77]

- Medications. This fix may bring a good sleep but downsides are many: cost, addiction, dependence, and side effects, one of which could be obesity. Also know that other medications can contain stimulants that may disrupt sleep.

- Limit caffeine. Know where it is: coffee, tea, sodas, and dark chocolate. Avoid any source too late in the day.

- Bedtime snack. Carbohydrates will enhance serotonin action, which helps with sleep. A piece of fruit, yogurt, or graham crackers are good choices.

- Get catch-up sleep. Let the kids sleep in on the weekends. Join them.

- Melatonin. Crossing many time zones is the fastest way to throw your inner clocks into a tizzy. Melatonin can help correct frazzled sleep-wake rhythms. Start with a low dose.

- The insalubrious effects of technology may be shifting as business, public organizations, and universities explore new applications so they, in the words of Google's founders, "don't be evil." New exercise games including Dance Dance Revolution and Wii Sports may counteract some damage. "Energy expended during active video game play was comparable to light or moderate exercise."[78] According to a recent review, many educational games teach nutrition and diet. Examples are *MyPyramid Blast-off Game* and *The Restaurant*. A recent Canadian review of 34 studies showed benefit from gaming by increasing both exercise and nutritional knowledge. The interesting analysis pointed to potential for video games in promoting healthy behaviors.[79] Use the new generation of gaming and social media to encourage healthy eating and exercise. *Farmville* from Zynga, Inc., has a new template to combat obesity. Buy a Fitbit or similar gadget to track your activity, calories, sleep, and weight.

- Social media can be a solution too. Temple University in Philadelphia tested a Facebook weight management intervention at their school. For eight weeks, 52 students were randomly assigned to one of three groups: Facebook (videos and other health tips sent online); Facebook Plus (which added text messaging and personalized feedback to the first); or control (received no intervention). The mostly female students were also racially diverse. At eight weeks, the Facebook Plus group had more weight loss than either plain Facebook or control, which was about the same. All of the participants said they would recommend the program to others. Because young people already are heavy users of social media, it may be one answer in combatting obesity.[80]

- Deal with worry. A Swedish study revealed significant links between sleep problems and concern about money and relationships.[81] That probably didn't need a study.

- Bright light therapy may be useful in reducing night eating. But light at night is also being questioned as a factor in increased breast cancer rates by researcher Barbra Dickerman and her colleagues who have reviewed compelling evidence and implications in female night-shift workers.[82]

- Cognitive therapy for insomnia or night eating. One study had 25 patients undergo ten sessions of cognitive behavior therapy. "[The] number of awakenings per week, depressed mood, and quality of life all improved."[83]

- Rediscover nature. Plants clean our lungs, animals comfort us, and an afternoon in a forest or at the beach calms us. Our place in the universe becomes apparent. So why do we increasingly avoid the outdoors? Germs, bears, poison ivy, fatigue, mud, sunburn, poor footwear, no phone signal, no time, chance of rain, too hot, too cold . . . all valid perhaps but still not enough to miss out on munificent nature. Take a page from the German school guide, which puts the smallest toddlers outdoors rain and shine. They sleep well.

It's all so simple. Humans have strayed far from the normal rhythms of biology. Modernity whether in the form of an iPad, fluorescent-lit cubicle, or a red-eye flight has robbed us of sleep and upset our inner clocks, our exquisitely timed network of genes, neurons, hormones, peptides, and even more we haven't discovered yet. What took millions of years to perfect is under siege and struggling to adapt. Gaining weight is a symptom of that distress.

Now go to bed. Without your phone.

AFTERWORD

. . . .

OBESITY IS MORE THAN TOO MANY SECOND helpings. For far too long we have asked individuals to summon the willpower to eat less and exercise more, all the while ignoring how modern life has created a massing cloud of obesogens.

The world we live in would astound and frighten our hunter-gatherer ancestors.

We air-condition offices—even in Alaska—so computers can breathe, we trade gym class for extra math, and we move to the suburbs for cherished extra space. Many good intentions paved the way to obesity.

Less-noble goals also permeate our world: cattle are fed growth hormones and antibiotics to increase profits, strong medications allow shorter but more visits for doctors and windfalls for drug firms, and cesarean sections suit our schedules but rob our newborns of a mother's unique microbial map.

If progress looks in the mirror, it won't be pretty: smart and comfortable, for sure, but with the added weight of a chronic disease called obesity, which threatens the health of our fragile ever-expanding planet.

Poor countries have more to lose. The rapid switch from hunger to obesity is alarming but should not have been a surprise. In a world fused closer by the day and hungry for the slickly marketed trends, rich countries have been exporting more than smartphones and sneakers.

Multinational firms flood the global marketplace with obesogenic products. Sales of soft drinks have doubled in the past decade, much of that rise coming from poor nations. Air-conditioning units cling to the most bereft apartment blocks. Cars outsell bicycles as incomes rise. Medications pour into bodies and water supplies. Guns replace fists, and people are scared to go outside.

Struggling nations buy up cheap oils and sugars to mimic their rich neighbors, yet they can ill-afford the high cost of obesity. Diabetes care alone threatens to consume much of their scant resources. One of the biggest tests for developing countries will be reconciling food insecurity and obesity, dangerous conspirators challenging global health.

As I was writing this book, new information came in at a dizzying pace. No sooner was one chapter finished than it was time to update another. The good news is that far more attention is being paid to this epidemic. Obesity commanded an entire conference at the United Nations in 2011; Mayor Bloomberg tried to ban large sodas in New York City the following year (grabbing headlines if not support); and chain restaurants scrambled to label menus before a 2013 deadline. Bisphenol A is being expelled from baby bottles, cities are carving out bike trails, and high-fructose corn syrup is reaching pariah status.

Still the food and beverage industry is treading on mixed messages. Will consumers buy healthy or not? Will they pay more for organic foods? As a result, companies hedge their bets by selling it all: bran flakes next to cocoa puffs; fruit juice next to cola; apple slices alongside fries. To their credit, global food companies, sensing a coming shift in consumer preferences and government policies, have pledged to remove 1.5 trillion calories from their products by 2015.

There are other signs of team effort.

Employers, such as Safeway, are rewarding lean workers with lower healthcare premiums. Others like Microsoft offer on-site gyms, pools, and basketball courts. And Google put a portion meter on free M&M dispensers dotting its offices.

Countries are waking up too. Mexico is cutting sugar and fat from school menus and feeding programs.[1] The United Kingdom is bringing cooking lessons into schools.[2] The United Arab Emirates has a sustainable car-free city in the works, expected to be operational by 2020.[3]

It's a start. But everyone—and that includes me, you, schools, banks, hospitals, restaurants, cities, and nations—must invest in turning this epidemic around. It can be done.

We need back-to-the-future moments. Whether allowing the body to adjust to seasonal warmth without air conditioners, treating sadness with strenuous exercise instead of strong antidepressants, eating beans and berries instead of chips and cheese fries, or replacing hard plastic containers with clay pots, the first goal is to simply unravel the long list of modern ways that turned out to be harmful.

Society needs to step up. That means governments, employers, insurers, and beyond. Bring back water fountains and open windows. Hold insurance and pharmaceutical companies to higher standards. Weave exercise into the workplace and bring it back into schools. Reduce premiums for preventive practices and subsidize healthy living by cutting prices of nutritious foods and yoga classes. Hundreds of ideas from innovators were tossed around in previous pages. When strategies prove successful, they should flow easily across borders, allowing every human being regardless of income to share in solutions for better health.

One out of four people on our planet is overweight or obese. Many shifts in our environment caused *globesity* and now much must be done to reverse it.

The species that endures is not afraid to change.

NOTES

. . . .

INTRODUCTION

1. "Adult Obesity Facts," Center for Disease Control and Prevention, accessed February 2013, http://www.cdc.gov/obesity/data/adult.html.

2. "Obesity and Overweight," World Health Organization, accessed February 2013, http://www.who.int/mediacentre/factsheets/fs311/en/index.html.

3. "Fact Sheet: Metabolic and Bariatric Surgery," American Society for Metabolic & Bariatric Surgery, accessed February 2013, http://s3.amazonaws.com/publicASMBS/Resources/Fact-Sheets/Metabolic-Bariatric-Surgery-Fact-Sheet-ASMBS2012.pdf.

4. G. Danaei et al., "The Preventable Causes of Death in the United States: Comparative Risk Assessment of Dietary, Lifestyle, and Metabolic Risk Factors," *Public Library of Science Medicine* 6, no. 4 (April 28, 2009).

5. "World Health Statistics," World Health Organization, accessed February 2013, http://www.who.int/gho/publications/world_health_statistics/EN_WHS2012_Full.pdf.

6. K. M. Flegal et al., "Association of All-Cause Mortality with Overweight and Obesity Using Standard Body Mass Index Categories: A Systematic Review and Meta-Analysis," *Journal of the American Medical Association* 309, no. 1 (January 2, 2013): 71–82. doi:10.1001.

7. E. A. Finkelstein et al., "Annual Medical Spending Attributable to Obesity: Payer- and Service-Specific Estimates," *Health Affairs* 28, no. 5 (2009): w822-w831.

8. "Diabetes Atlas," International Diabetes Federation, idf.org/diabetesatlas.

9. "Latest Diabetes Figures Paint Grim Global Picture," October 18, 2009, http://www.idf.org/latest-diabetes-figures-paint-grim-global-picture.

10. "Healthcare Leaders United to Fight Diabetes Epidemic," International Diabetes Federation, April 16, 2012, www.idf.org/healthcare-leaders-unite-fight-diabetes-epidemic.

11. "Are Americans Ready to Solve the Weight of the Nation?" Johns Hopkins Bloomberg School of Public Health, August 1, 2012, http://www.jhsph.edu/news/news-releases/2012/barry-weight-attitudes.html.

12. International Diabetes Federation, "Diabetes in the Young" http://www.idf.org/diabetesatlas/5e/diabetes-in-the-young.

13. "About Obesity," Public Health England, http://www.noo.org.uk/NOO_about_obesity/child_obesity/UK_prevalence.

14. S. W. Ng et al., "The Prevalence and Trends of Overweight, Obesity and Nutrition-Related Non-Communicable Diseases in the Arabian Gulf States," *Obesity Reviews* 12, no. 1 (January 2011): 1–13, http://www.ncbi.nlm.nih.gov/pubmed/20546144

15. "Excerpt: Dean Ornish's 'The Spectrum,'" ABC News, January 3, 2007, http://abcnews.go.com/GMA/PersonalBest/story?id=4077021&page=10.

16. M. A. Subramanyam et al., "Is Economic Growth Associated with Reduction in Child Undernutrition in India?" *PLoS Med* 8, no. 3 (March 8, 2011): e1000424. doi: 10.1371/journal.pmed.1000424, http://www.plosmedicine.org/article/info%3Adoi%2F10.1371%2Fjournal.pmed.1000424.

17. Frank B. Hu, *Obesity Epidemiology* (New York: Oxford University Press, 2008).

18. M. A. Cornier, "Is Your Brain to Blame for Weight Regain?" *Physiology & Behavior* 104, no. 4 (Sept. 26, 2011): 608–12. doi: 10.1016.

19. E. J. McAllister et al., "Ten Putative Contributors to the Obesity Epidemic," *Critical Reviews in Food Science & Nutrition* 49, no. 10 (November 2009): 868–913.

CHAPTER 1

1. "LG Solidifies Its Leadership in Middle East Air Conditioning Market with New Production Facility in Saudi Arabia," LG Electronics, accessed February 2013, http://www.lg.com/us/press-release/lg-solidifies-its-leadership-in-middle-east-air-conditioning-market-with-new-production-facility-in-saudi-arabia.

2. The thermoneutral zone (TNZ) is the range of ambient temperature in which energy expenditure is not required for homeothermy. Exposure to ambient temperatures above or below the TNZ increases energy expenditure and decreases energy stores (that is, fat).

3. A. A. Mahfouz et al., "Obesity and Related Behaviors among Adolescent School Boys in Abha City, Southwestern Saudi Arabia," *Journal of Tropical Pediatrics* 54, no. 2 (April 2008): 120–24.

4. F. al-Mahroos and K. al-Roomi, "Overweight and Obesity in the Arabian Peninsula: An Overview," *Journal of the Royal Society for the Promotion of Health* 119, no. 4 (December 1999): 251–53.

5. A. I. Ismail, A. H. al-Abdulwahab, and A. S. al-Mulhim, "Osteoarthritis of Knees and Obesity in Eastern Saudi Arabia," *Saudi Medical Journal* 27, no. 11 (November 2006): 1742–4.

6. D. R. Bassett, P. L. Schneider, and G. E. Huntington, "Physical Activity in an Old Order Amish Community," *Medicine & Science in Sports & Exercise* 36, no. 8 (August 2004):1447.

7. Gavin Weightman, *Frozen Water Trade: A True Story* (New York: Hyperion, 2004).

8. Henry Miller, *The Air-Conditioned Nightmare* (New York: New Directions, 1970).

9. Adam Rome, *The Bulldozer in the Countryside: Suburban Sprawl and the Rise of American Environmentalism* (Cambridge University Press, 2001).

10. "Fact Sheet." United Technologies Corporation, accessed February 2013, http://www.carrier.com/carrier/en/worldwide/about/fact-sheet.

11. William Saletan, "A/C D.C.: The Deluded World of Air Conditioning," *Slate*, August 5, 2006, accessed February 2013, http://www.slate.com/articles/health_and_science/human_nature/2006/08/ac_dc.html.

12. Stan Cox, "Cooling a Warming Planet: A Global Air Conditioning Surge," Yale Environment 360, July 10, 2012, accessed February 2013, http://e360.yale.edu/feature/cooling_a_warming_planet_a_global_air_conditioning_surge/2550.

13. "Air Conditioning: No Sweat," *The Economist*, January 5, 2013, http://www.economist.com/news/international/21569017-artificial-cooling-makes-hot-places-bearablebut-worryingly-high-cost-no-sweat.

14. James Fergusson, "A Brief History of Air-Conditioning," *Prospect*, September 24, 2006, accessed February 2013, http://www.prospectmagazine.co.uk/magazine/abriefhistoryofairconditioning.

15. Cox, "Cooling a Warming Planet: A Global Air Conditioning."

16. C. P. Herman, "Effects of Heat on Appetite," in B. M. Marriott, ed., *Nutritional Needs in Hot Environments: Applications for Military Personnel in Field Operations* (National Academy Press: Washington DC, 1993), 187–214.

17. J. W. West, "Effects of Heat Stress on Production in Dairy Cattle," *Journal of Dairy Science* 86, no. 6 (June 2003): 2131–44.

18. R. J. Collier, G. E. Dahl, and M. J. VanBaale, "Major Advances Associated with Environmental Effects on Dairy Cattle," *Journal of Dairy Science* 89, no. 4 (April 2006): 1244–53.

19. J. M. Fletcher, "Effects on Growth and Endocrine Status of Maintaining Obese and Lean Zucker Rats at 22°C and 30°C from Weaning," *Physiology & Behavior* 37, no. 4 (1986): 597–602.

20. C. J. De Souza and A. H. Meier, "Alterations in Body Fat Stores and Plasma Insulin Levels with Daily Intervals of Heat Exposure in Holtzman Rats," *American Journal of Physiology* 265, no. 5, pt. 2 (November 1993): R1109–14.

21. S. E. Evans and D. L. Ingram, "The Effect of Ambient Temperature upon the Secretion of Thyroxine in the Young Pig," *Journal of Physiology* 264, no. 2 (January): 511–21.

22. M. S. Westerterp-Plantenga et al., "Energy Metabolism in Humans at a Lowered Ambient Temperature," *European Journal of Clinical Nutrition* 56, no. 4 (April 2002): 288–96.

23. Frank B. Hu, *Obesity Epidemiology* (New York: Oxford University Press, 2008).

24. S. M. Bouali et al., "Influence of Ambient Temperature on the Effects of NPY on Body Temperature and Food Intake," *Pharmacology, Biochemistry &*

Behavior 50, no. 3 (March 1995): 473–75.

25. Ueno T, Ohnaka T, "Influence of Long-Term Exposure to an Air-Conditioned Environment on the Diurnal Cortisol Rhythm," *Journal of Physiological Anthropology* 25, no. 6 (November 2006): 357–62.

26. C. L. White et al., "Effect of a High or Low Ambient Perinatal Temperature on Adult Obesity on Osborne-Mendel and S5B/PI Rats," *American Journal of Physiology: Regulatory, Integrative and Comparative Physiology* 288, no. 5 (May 2005): R1376-84.

27. "The Caveman's Curse," in "Special Report: Obesity," *The Economist* (December 15, 2012): 3–16.

28. A. S. Kauffman, A. Cabrera, and I. Zucker, "Energy Intake and Fur in Summer- and Winter-Acclimated Siberian Hamsters (*Phosphorus sungorus*)," *American Journal of Physiology - Regulatory, Integrative and Comparative Physiology* 281, no. 2 (August 2001): R519–27.

29. D. B. Downey and H. R. Boughton, "Childhood Body Mass Index Gain during the Summer Versus during the School Year," *New Directions for Youth Development* 114 (Summer 2007): 33–43.

30. A. L. Carrel, "School-Based Fitness Changes Are Lost during the Summer Vacation," *Archives of Pediatrics & Adolescent Medicine* 161, no. 6 (June 2007): 561–64.

31. Kobayashi M, Kobayashi M, "The Relationship between Obesity and Seasonal Variation in Body Weight among Elementary School Children in Tokyo," *Economics & Human Biology* 4, no. 2 (June 2006): 253–61.

32. Fergusson, "A Brief History of Air-Conditioning."

33. "Air Conditioning: No Sweat," *The Economist*, January 5, 2013.

34. R. J. Collier, G. E. Dahl, and M. J. VanBaale, "Major Advances Associated with Environmental Effects on Dairy Cattle," *Journal of Dairy Science* 89, no. 4 (April 2006): 1244–53.

35. S. L. Wijers et al., "Recent Advances in Adaptive Thermogenesis: Potential Implications for the Treatment of Obesity," *Obesity Reviews* 10, no. 2 (March 2009): 218–26. doi: 10.1111/j.1467-789X.2008.00538.x, emphasis added.

36. Michael Tortorello, "Bringing in the Big Fans," *New York Times* Online (June 16, 2011), http://www.nytimes.com/2011/06/16/garden/bringing-in-the-big-fans.html?pagewanted=1&ref=garden

37. Rim D. Coder, "Identified Benefits of Community Trees and Forests," October 1996 (University of Georgia), http://www.marshalltrees.com/upload /articles_files/art_31attached_file.pdf.

CHAPTER 2

1. "Drug Ratings for ACTOS," Askapatient.com, accessed March 4, 2013, http://www.askapatient.com/viewrating.asp?drug=21073&name=ACTOS.

2. "The Use of Medicines in the United States: Review of 2011," IMS

Institute for Healthcare Informatics, April 2012, accessed March 4, 2013, http://www.imshealth.com/ims/Global/Content/Insights/IMS%20Institute%20for%20Healthcare%20Informatics/IHII_Medicines_in_U.S_Report_2011.pdf.

3. W. S. Leslie, C. R. Hankey, and M. E. Lean, "Weight Gain As an Adverse Effect of Some Commonly Prescribed Drugs: A Systematic Review," *Quarterly Journal of Medicine* 100, no. 7 (July 2007): 395–404.

4. Q. Gu, C. F. Dillon, and Vivki L. Burt, "NCHS Data Brief," no. 42 (September 2010), accessed March 3, 2013, http://www.cdc.gov/nchs/data/databriefs/db42.htm.

5. "2011 National Diabetes Fact Sheet," Centers for Disease Control and Prevention (CDC), http://www.cdc.gov/diabetes/pubs/factsheet11.htm.

6. J. E. Shaw, R. A. Sicree, and P. Z. Zimmet, "Global Estimates of the Prevalence of Diabetes for 2010 and 2030," *Diabetes Research & Clinical Practice* 87, no. 1 (January 2010): 4–14

7. Centers for Disease Control and Prevention, "Health, United States, 2009," cdc.gov/data/hus/hus09.pdf, p. 94.

8. American Diabetes Association, "Economic Costs of Diabetes in the U.S. in 2012," March 6, 2013, http://care.diabetesjournals.org/content/early/2013/03/05/dc12-2625.full.pdf; "Economic Costs of Diabetes in the US in 2007," *Diabetes Care* 31 (2008): 1–20. doi: 10.2337/dc08-S001.

9. "The Use of Medicines in the United States: Review of 2011," IMS Institute for Healthcare Informatics, April 2012.

10. P. Zhang et al., "Global Healthcare Expenditure on Diabetes for 2010 and 2030" *Diabetes Research and Clinical Practice* 87, no. 3 (March 2010): 293–301, accessed March 4, 2013, http://www.idf.org/webdata/docs/PIIS0168822710000495.pdf.

11. E. J. McAllister et al., "Ten Putative Contributors to the Obesity Epidemic," *Critical Reviews in Food Science & Nutrition* 49, no. 10 (November 2009): 868–913.

12. D. C. Simonson et al., "Efficacy, Safety, and Dose-Response Characteristics of Glipizide Gastrointestinal Therapeutic System on Glycaemic Control and Insulin Secretion in NIDDM: Results of Two Multicenter, Randomized, Placebo-Controlled Trials," *Diabetes Care* 20, no. 4 (April 1997): 597–606.

13. P. Segal et al., "The Efficacy and Safety of Miglitol Therapy Compared with Glibenclamide in Patients with NIDDM Inadequately Controlled by Diet Alone," *Diabetes Care* 20, no. 5 (May 1997): 687–91.

14. McAllister et al., "Ten Putative Contributors to the Obesity Epidemic."

15. A. Lund and F. K. Knop, "Worry vs. Knowledge About Treatment-Associated Hypoglycemia and Weight Gain in Type 2 Diabetic Patients on Metformin and/or Sulphonylurea," *Current Medical Research & Opinion* 28, no. 5 (May 2012): 731–36.

16. McAllister et al., "Ten Putative Contributors to the Obesity Epidemic."

17. J. Q. Purnell and C. Weyer, "Weight Effect of Current and Experimental

Drugs for Diabetes Mellitus: From Promotion to Alleviation of Obesity," *Treatments in Endocrinology* 2, no. 1 (2003): 33–47.

18. S. S. Schwartz and B. A. Kohl, "Glycemic Control and Weight Reduction Without Causing Hypoglycemia: The Case for Continued Safe Aggressive Care of Patients with Type 2 Diabetes Mellitus and Avoidance of Therapeutic Inertia," *Mayo Clinic Proceedings* 85, no. 12 suppl. (December 2010): S15–26.

19. R. A. DeFronzo et al., "ACT NOW Study. Pioglitazone for Diabetes Prevention in Impaired Glucose Tolerance," *New England Journal of Medicine* 364, no. 12 (March 24, 2011): 1104–15.

20. R. A. DeFronzo and M. Abdul-Ghani, "Type 2 Diabetes Can Be Prevented with Early Pharmacological Intervention," *Diabetes Care* 24, no. 34, suppl. 2 (May 2011): S202–9.

21. Centers for Disease Control and Prevention, "National Diabetes Fact Sheet: National Estimates and General Information on Diabetes and Prediabetes in the United States, 2011" (Atlanta: U.S. Department of Health and Human Services, Centers for Disease Control and Prevention, 2011), accessed March 4, 2013, http://www.cdc.gov/diabetes/pubs/pdf/ndfs_2011.pdf.

22. C. L. Gillies et al., "Pharmacological and Lifestyle Interventions to Prevent or Delay Type 2 Diabetes in People with Impaired Glucose Tolerance: Systematic Review and Meta-Analysis," *British Medical Journal* 334, no. 7588 (February 2007): 299.

23. J. L. Chiasson, M. C. Brindisi, and R. Rabasa-Lhoret, "The Prevention of Type 2 Diabetes: What Is the Evidence?" *Minerva Endocrinology* 30, no. 3 (September 2005): 179–91.

24. H. E. Bays, R. H. Chapman, and S. Grandy, "The Relationship of Body Mass Index to Diabetes Mellitus, Hypertension and Dyslipidemia: Comparison of Data from Two National Surveys," *International Journal of Clinical Practice* 61, no. 5 (May 2007: 737–47.

25. S. Klein et al., "American Diabetes Association, North American Association for the Study of Obesity, American Society for Clinical Nutrition Weight Management through Lifestyle Modification for the Prevention and Management of Type 2 Diabetes: Rationale and Strategies: A Statement of the American Diabetes Association, the North American Association for the Study of Obesity, and the American Society for Clinical Nutrition," *Diabetes Care* 27, no. 8 (August 2004): 2067–73.

26. J. B. Dixon et al., "Bariatric Surgery: An IDF Statement for Obese Type 2 Diabetes," *Diabetic Medicine* 28, no. 6 (June 2011): 628–42. doi: 10.1111/j.1464-5491.2011.03306.x

27. "The Use of Medicines in the United States: Review of 2011," IMS Institute for Healthcare Informatics, April 2012.

28. Ibid.

29. C. Mastronardi et al., "Long-Term Body Weight Outcomes of Antidepressant–Environment Interactions," *Molecular Psychiatry* 16, no. 3 (March 2011): 265–72.

30. McAllister et al., "Ten Putative Contributors to the Obesity Epidemic."

31. S. A. Montgomery, P. E. Reimitz, and M. Zivkov, "Mirtazapine versus Amitriptyline in the Long-Term Treatment of Depression: A Double-Blind Placebo-Controlled Study," *International Clinical Psychopharmacology* 13, no. 2 (March 1998): 63–73.

32. S. Caproni et al., "Migraine Preventive Drug-Induced Weight Gain May Be Mediated by Effects on Hypothalamic Peptides: The Results of a Pilot Study," *Cephalalgia* 31, no. 5 (April 2011): 543–49. doi: 10.1177/0333102410392605.

33. M. Fava et al., "Fluoxetine Versus Sertraline and Paroxetine in Major Depressive Disorder: Changes in Weight with Long-Term Treatment," *Journal Clinical Psychiatry* 61, no. 11 (November 2000): 863–67.

34. N. Sussman, D. L. Ginsberg, J. Bikoff, "Effects of Nefazodone on Body Weight: A Pooled Analysis of Selective Serotonin Reuptake Inhibitor- and Imipramine-Controlled Trials," *Journal Clinical Psychiatry* 62, no. 4 (April 2001): 256–60.

35. R. Ness-Abramof and C. M. Apovian, "Drug-Induced Weight Gain," *Drugs of Today* (Barcelona, Spain) 41, no. 8 (August 2005): 547–55.

36. Sussman, Ginsberg, and Bikoff, "Effects of Nefazodone on Body Weight."

37. H. Croft et al., "Effect on Body Weight of Bupropion Sustained-Release in Patients with Major Depression Treated for 52 Weeks," *Clinical Therapeutics* 24, no. 4 (April 2002): 662–72.

38. Jonathan Rottenberg, "Charting the Depth: Reflections on the Science of Depression," Psychology Today, July 23, 2010, accessed March 5, 2013, http://www.psychologytoday.com/blog/charting-the-depths/201007/the-serotonin-theory-depression-is-collapsing.

39. Mastronardi et al., "Long-Term Body Weight Outcomes of Antidepressant–Environment Interactions."

40. McAllister et al., "Ten Putative Contributors to the Obesity Epidemic."

41. "The Use of Medicines," IMS Institute for Healthcare Informatics.

42. Robert Whitaker, *Anatomy of an Epidemic: Magic Bullets, Psychiatric Drugs, and the Astonishing Rise of Mental Illness in America* (New York: Crown, 2010).

43. "America's State of Mind: A Report by Medco," Medco Health Solutions, accessed September 22, 20113, http://apps.who.int/medicinedocs/documents/s19032en/s19032en.pdf.

44. R. Ganguli, "Weight gain associated with antipsychotic drugs," *Journal Clinical Psychiatry* 60, suppl. 21 (1999): 20–24.

45. A. H. Barnett et al., "Minimising Metabolic and Cardiovascular Risk in Schizophrenia: Diabetes, Obesity and Dyslipidaemia," *Journal of Psychopharmacology* 21, no. 4 (June 2007): 357–73.

46. D. B. Allison et al., "Antipsychotic-Induced Weight Gain: A Comprehensive Research Synthesis," *American Journal of Psychiatry* 156, no. 11 (November 1999): 1686–96.

47. D. C. Henderson et al., "Clozapine, Diabetes Mellitus, Weight Gain, and Lipid Abnormalities: A Five-Year Naturalistic Study," *American Journal of Psychiatry* 157, no. 6 (June 2000): 975–81.

48. G. Jassim et al., "Acute Effects of Orexigenic Antipsychotic Drugs on Lipid and Carbohydrate Metabolism in Rats," *Psychopharmacology* (Berlin, Germany) 219, no. 3 (February 2012): 783–94.

49. R. B. Zipursky et al., "Course and Predictors of Weight Gain in People with First-Episode Psychosis Treated with Olanzapine or Haloperidol," *British Journal of Psychiatry* 187 (December 2005): 537–43.

50. F. M. Theisen et al., "Spectrum of Binge Eating Symptomatology in Patients Treated with Clozapine and Olanzapine," *Journal of Neural Transmission* 110, no. 1 (January 2003): 111–21.

51. D. Gothelf et al., "Weight Gain Associated with Increased Food Intake and Low Habitual Activity Levels in Male Adolescent Schizophrenic Inpatients Treated with Olanzapine," *American Journal of Psychiatry* 159, no. 6 (June 2002): 1055–57.

52. T. Brömel et al., "Serum Leptin Levels Increase Rapidly after Initiation of Clozapine Therapy," *Molecular Psychiatry* 3, no. 1 (January 1998): 76–80.

53. E. Stip et al., "Neural Changes Associated with Appetite Information Processing in Schizophrenic Patients after 16 Weeks of Olanzapine Treatment," *Translational Psychiatry* 2, no. e128 (June 2012). doi: 10.1038/tp.2012.53.

54. V. L. Albaugh et al., "Olanzapine Promotes Fat Accumulation in Male Rats by Decreasing Physical Activity, Repartitioning Energy and Increasing Adipose Tissue Lipogenesis While Impairing Lipolysis," *Molecular Psychiatry* 16, no. 5 (May 2011): 569–81.

55. Syed Ahmer, Rashid A. M. Khan, and Saleem Perwaiz Iqbal, "Association between Antipsychotics and Weight Gain among Psychiatric Outpatients in Pakistan: A Retrospective Cohort Study," *Annals of General Psychiatry* 7, no. 12 (2008). doi:10.1186/1744-859X-7-12.

56. Ibid.

57. Ibid.

58. Barnett et al., "Minimising Metabolic and Cardiovascular Risk in Schizophrenia."

59. V. Woo, S. B. Harris, R. L. Houlden, "Canadian Diabetes Association Position Paper: Antipsychotic Medications and Associated Risks of Weight Gain and Diabetes," *Canadian Journal of Diabetes* 29 (2005): 111–12.

60. A. Cimo et al., "Effective Lifestyle Interventions to Improve Type II Diabetes Self-Management for Those with Schizophrenia or Schizoaffective Disorder: A Systematic Review" *BioMed Central Psychiatry* 12, no. 2 (March 2012): 24. doi: 10.1186/1471-244X-12-24.

61. A. Ströhle, "Physical activity, exercise, depression and anxiety disorders," *Journal of Neural Transmission* 116, no. 6 (June 2009): 777–84.

62. P. J. Carek, S. E. Laibstain, S. M. Carek, "Exercise for the Treatment of

Depression and Anxiety," *International Journal of Psychiatry in Medicine* 41, no. 1 (2011): 15–28.

63. D. Tordeurs et al., "Effectiveness of Physical Exercise in Psychiatry: A Therapeutic Approach?" *Encephale* 37, no. 5 (October 2011): 345–52. doi: 10.1016/j.encep.2011.02.003.

64. Robert Whitaker, *Anatomy of an Epidemic* (New York: Crown, 2010).

65. V. Butterweck, "Mechanism of Action of St John's Wort in Depression: What Is Known?" *CNS Drugs* 17, no. 8 (2003): 539–62.

66. J. Sirven, "Prescription Medications that Make You Gain Weight," April 29, 2013, http://nbclatino.com/2013/04/29/prescription-medications-that-make-you-gain-weight; E. Ben-Menachem, "Weight Issues for People with Epilepsy—A Review," *Epilepsia* 48 (suppl. 9): 42–45.

67. Ness-Abramof and Apovian, "Drug-Induced Weight Gain."

68. T. Baptista et al., "Lithium and Body Weight Gain," *Pharmacopsychiatry* 28, no. 2 (March 1995): 35–44.

69. A. Sharma et al., "Beta-Adrenergic Receptor Blockers and Weight Gain: A Systematic Analysis," *Hypertension* 37, no. 2 (February 2001): 250–54.

70. Ibid.

71. F. M. Sacks et al., "Effects on Blood Pressure of Reduced Dietary Sodium and the Dietary Approaches to Stop Hypertension (DASH) Diet," *New England Journal of Medicine* 344 (January 4, 2001): 3–10.

72. Z. Y. Chen et al., "Anti-Hypertensive Nutraceuticals and Functional Foods," *Journal of Agricultural and Food Chemistry* 57, no. 11 (June 10, 2009): 4485–99.

73. L. S. Pescatello et al., "American College of Sports Medicine Position Stand. Exercise and Hypertension," *Medicine & Science in Sports & Exercise* 36, no. 3 (March 2004): 533–53.

74. S. P. Whelton et al., "Effect of Aerobic Exercise on Blood Pressure: A Meta-Analysis of Randomized, Controlled Trials," *Annals of Internal Medicine* 136, no. 7 (April 2, 2002): 493–503.

75. N. R. Okonta, "Does Yoga Therapy Reduce Blood Pressure in Patients with Hypertension? An Integrative Review," *Holistic Nursing Practice* 26, no. 3 (May–June 2012): 137–41.

76. R. B. Stricker and B. Goldberg, "Weight Gain Associated with Protease Inhibitor Therapy in HIV-Infected Patients," *Research in Virology* 149, no. 2 (March–April 1998): 123–26.

77. R. J. Kim and R. M. Rutstein, "Impact of Antiretroviral Therapy on Growth, Body Composition and Metabolism in Pediatric HIV Patients," *Paediatric Drugs* 12, no. 3 (June 2010): 187–99.

78. D. Signorini et al., "What Should We Know About Metabolic Syndrome and Lipodystrophy in AIDS?" *Revista da Associação Médica Brasileira* 58, no. 1 (January–February 2013): 70–75. Retrieved May 31, 2012,

79. I. Yoshikawa et al., "Long-Term Treatment with Proton Pump Inhibitor

Is Associated with Undesired Weight Gain," *World Journal of Gastroenterology* 15, no. 38 (October 14, 2009): 4794–98.

80. B. C. Jacobson et al., "Body-Mass Index and Symptoms of Gastroesophageal Reflux in Women," *New England Journal of Medicine* 354 (June 1, 2006): 2340–48.

81. M. F. Prummel et al., "Randomized Double Blind Trial of Prednisone Versus Radiotherapy in Graves' Ophthalmopathy," *Lancet* 342, no. 8877 (October 16, 1993): 949–54.

82. M. F. Gallo et al., "Combination contraceptives: effects on weight," *Cochrane Database of Systematic Reviews* no. 9 (September 2011):CD003987.

83. E. Espey et al., "Depo-Provera Associated with Weight Gain in Navajo Women," *Contraception* 62, no. 2 (August 2000): 55–58.

84. L. Aronne, "A Practical Guide to Drug-Induced Weight Gain," in L. Aronne, ed., *Drug-Induced Weight Gain: Non-CNS Medications* (Minneapolis: McGraw-Hill, 2002), 77–91.

85. J. Ratliff et al., "Association of Prescription H1 Antihistamine Use with Obesity: Results from the National Health and Nutrition Examination Survey," *Obesity* (Silver Spring, MD) 18, no. 12 (December 2010): 2398–2400.

CHAPTER 3

1. F. Grün and B. Blumberg, "Environmental Obesogens: Organotins and Endocrine Disruption via Nuclear Receptor Signaling," *Endocrinology* 147, no. 6 suppl (June 2006): S50–55.

2. P. F. Baillie-Hamilton, "Chemical Toxins: A Hypothesis to Explain the Global Obesity Epidemic," *Journal of Alternative & Complementary Medicine* 8, no. 2 (April 2002): 185–92.

3. Ibid.

4. R. R. Newbold, "Impact of Environmental Endocrine Disrupting Chemicals on the Development of Obesity," *Hormones* (Athens) 9, no. 3 (July–September 2010): 206–17, www.hormones.gr/692/article/article.html.

5. Buck Levin, *Environmental Nutrition: Understanding the Link between Environment, Food Quality, and Disease* (HingePin Integrative Learning Materials, 1999).

6. R. J. Kavlock et. al, 1996 "Research Needs for the Risk Assessment of Health and Environmental Effects of Endocrine Disruptors," *Environmental Health Perspectives* 104 (suppl. 4): 715–40, in P. Alonso-Magdalena et al., "Bisphenol-A: A New Diabetogenic Factor?" *Hormones* 9, no. 2 (2010): 118–26.

7. M. A. Elobeid and D. B. Allison, "Putative Environmental-Endocrine Disruptors and Obesity: A Review," *Current Opinion in Endocrinology, Diabetes & Obesity* 15, no. 5 (October 2008): 403–8. doi: 10.1097/MED.0b013e32830ce95c.

8. F. Grün, "Obesogens," *Current Opinion in Endocrinology, Diabetes & Obesity* 17, no. 5 (October 2010): 453–59.

9. L. N. Vandenberg et al., "Hormones and Endocrine-Disrupting Chemicals: Low-Dose Effects and Nonmonotonic Dose Responses," *Endocrine Reviews* 33, no. 3 (June 2012): 378–455.

10. F. Grün and B. Blumberg, "Endocrine Disrupters As Obesogens," *Molecular and Cellular Endocrinology* 304, no. 1–2 (May 25, 2009): 19–29.

11. B. S. Rubin et al., "Perinatal Exposure to Low Doses of Bisphenol A Affects Body Weight, Patterns of Estrous Cyclicity, and Plasma LH Levels," *Environmental Health Perspectives* 109, no. 7 (July 2001): 675–80.

12. B. S. Rubin and A. Soto, "Bisphenol A: Perinatal Exposure and Body Weight," *Molecular and Cellular Endocrinology* 304, no. 1–3 (May 25, 2009): 55.

13. N. Blakar, "BPA Levels Tied to Obesity in Youths," *New York Times*, September 25, 2012, D6. See also L. Trasande, T. M. Attina, and J. Blustein, "Association between Urinary Bisphenol A Concentration and Obesity Prevalence in Children and Adolescents," *Journal of the American Medical Association* 308, no. 11 (September 19, 2012): 1113–21.

14. A. C. Farley et al., "Interventions for Preventing Weight Gain after Smoking Cessation, January 18, 2012, summaries.cochrane.org/CD006219/interventions-for-weight-gain-after-smoking-cessation.

15. R. J. Witorsch and J. A. Thomas, "Personal Care Products and Endocrine Disruption: A Critical Review of the Literature," *Critical Reviews in Toxicology* 40, suppl. 3 (November 2010): 1–30.

16. "Cosmetics," U.S. Food and Drug Administration, accessed December 5, 2010, updated September 3, 2013, http://www.fda.gov/Cosmetics/ProductandIngredientSafety/SelectedCosmeticIngredients/ucm128042.htm.

17. R. W. Stahlhut et al., "Concentrations of Urinary Phthalate Metabolites are Associated with Increased Waist Circumference and Insulin Resistance in Adult U.S. Males," *Environmental Health Perspectives* 115, no. 6 (June 2007): 876–82.

18. E. E. Hatch et al., "Association of Urinary Phthalate Metabolite Concentrations with Body Mass Index and Waist Circumference: A Cross-Sectional Study of NHANES Data, 1999–2002," *Environmental Health* 7 (2008): 27.

19. R. R. Newbold, "Impact of Environmental Endocrine Disrupting Chemicals on the Development of Obesity," *Hormones* (Athens) 9, no. 3 (July–September 2010): 206–17

20. Ibid.

21. Ibid.

22. L. Liu et al., "Effect of Bisphenol A Exposure during Early Development on Body Weight and Glucose Metabolism of Female Filial Rats," *Wei Sheng Yan Jiu* 41, no. 4 (July 2012): 543–45, 550.

23. T. I. Halldorsson et al., "Prenatal Exposure to Perfluorooctanoate and Risk of Overweight at 20 Years of Age: A Prospective Cohort Study," *Environmental Health Perspectives* 120, no. 5 (May 2012): 668–73.

24. K. S. Betts, "Perfluoroalkyl Acids: What Is the Evidence Telling Us?"

Environmental Health Perspectives 115, no. 5 (May 2007): A250–A256.

25. Grün and Blumberg, "Environmental Obesogens."

26. R. Chamorro-García et al., "Transgenerational Inheritance of Increased Fat Depot Size, Stem Cell Reprogramming, and Hepatic Steatosis Elicited by Prenatal Exposure to the Obesogen Tributyltin in Mice," *Environmental Health Perspectives* 121, no. 3 (March 2013): 359–66. doi: 10.1289/ehp.1205701.

27. S. D. Leary et al., "Smoking during Pregnancy and Offspring Fat and Lean Mass in Childhood," *Obesity* (Silver Spring, MD) 14, no. 12 (December 2006): 2284–93.

28. E. Oken, E. B. Levitan, M. W. Gillman, "Maternal Smoking during Pregnancy and Child Overweight: Systematic Review and Meta-Analysis," *International Journal of Obesity* (London) 32, no. 2 (February 2008): 201–210.

29. M. A. Mendez et al., "Maternal Smoking Very Early in Pregnancy Is Related to Child Overweight at Age 5–7 Y.," *American Journal of Clinical Nutrition* 87, no. 6 (June 2008): 1906–13.

30. Leary et al., "Smoking during Pregnancy."

31. V. T. Tong et al., "Age and Racial/Ethnic Disparities in Prepregnancy Smoking among Women Who Delivered Live Births," *Preventing Chronic Disease* 8, no. 6 (2011): A121.

32. Leary et al., "Smoking during Pregnancy."

33. "State of the Air 2012," American Lung Association, http://www.lung.org/associations/states/california/assets/pdfs/sota-2012/sota-2012-ca-report.pdf.

34. Kim Murphy, "Fairbanks Area, Trying to Stay Warm, Chokes on Wood Stove Pollution," *Los Angeles Times*, February 16, 2013.

35. "Global Health Observatory: Outdoor Air Pollution," World Health Organization, accessed March 8, 2013, http://www.who.int/gho/phe/outdoor_air_pollution/en.

36. Q. Sun et al., "Ambient Air Pollution Exaggerates Adipose Inflammation and Insulin Resistance in a Mouse Model of Diet-Induced Obesity," *Circulation* 119, no. 4 (February 3, 2009): 538–46.

37. J. F. Pearson et al., "Association between Fine Particulate Matter and Diabetes Prevalence in the U.S." *Diabetes Care* 33, no. 10 (October 2010): 2196–201.

38. "DDT and Its Derivatives," International Programme on Chemical Safety, accessed August 15, 2013, http://www.inchem.org/documents/ehc/ehc/ehc009.htm.

39. Agency for Toxic Substances and Disease Registry (ATSDR). Toxicological Profile for 4,4-DDT, 4,4-DDE, and 4,4-DDD. Public Health Service, U.S. Department of Health and Human Services, Atlanta, GA. 1994.

40. M. A. Mendez et al., "Prenatal Organochlorine Compound Exposure, Rapid Weight Gain, and Overweight in Infancy," *Environmental Health Perspectives* 119, no. 2 (February 2011): 272–78.

41. A. Smink et al., "Exposure to Hexachlorobenzene during Pregnancy

Increases the Risk of Overweight in Children Aged 6 Years," *Acta Paediatricia* 97, no. 10 (October 2008): 1465–69.

42. T. L. Lassiter et al., "Neonatal Exposure to Parathion Alters Lipid Metabolism in Adulthood: Interactions with Dietary Fat Intake and Implications for Neurodevelopmental Deficits," *Brain Research Bulletin* 81 (2010): 85-91.

43. Grün and Blumberg, "Environmental Obesogens."

44. D. Müllerová and J. Kopecký, "White Adipose Tissue: Storage and Effector Site for Environmental Pollutants," *Physiology Research* 56, no. 4 (2007): 375–81.

45. E. Dirinck et al., "Obesity and Persistent Organic Pollutants: Possible Obesogenic Effect of Organochlorine Pesticides and Polychlorinated Biphenyls," *Obesity* (Silver Spring, MD) 19, no. 4 (April 2011): 709–14.

46. "How does Safe Water Impact Global Health," World Health Organization, June 25, 2008, accessed March 9, 2013, http://www.who.int/features/qa/70/en.

47. David A. Fahrenthold, "Six Years Later, Gender-Bending Fish in Our Water Supply Remain a Mystery," *Washington Post*, November 24, 2009, http://articles.washingtonpost.com/2009-11-24/news/36901787_1_intersex-fish-male-fish-vicki-s-blazer.

48. Andrea Fuller, "Quality of Bottled Water Questioned in Congress," *New York Times*, July 8, 2009, accessed March 8, 2013, http://www.nytimes.com/2009/07/09/us/politics/09bottle.html?_r=0.

49. John Noble Wilford, "Roman Empire's Fall is Linked with Gout and Lead Poisoning," *New York Times*, March 17, 1983.

50. "Supplying Safe Drinking Water: Don't blame the Pill for Estrogen in Drinking Water" American Chemical Society, February 16, 2011, accessed April 22, 2013. http://www.acs.org/content/acs/en/pressroom/podcasts/global-challenges/drinkingwater/supplying-safe-drinking-water-dont-blame-the-pill-for-estrogen.html.

51. E. Zuccato et al., "Pharmaceuticals in the Environment in Italy: Causes, Occurrence, Effects and Control," *Environmental Science and Pollution Research International* 13, no. 1 (January 2006): 15–21.

52. R. C. Thompson et al., "Plastics, the Environment and Human Health: Current Consensus and Future Trends," *Philisophical Transactions of the Royal Society* 364, no. 1526 (July 27, 2009): 2153–66. doi: 10.1098/rstb.2009.0053.

53. "Can Birth Control Hormones Be Filtered from the Water Supply?" *Scientific American*, July 28, 2009, accessed March 9, 2013, http://www.scientificamerican.com/article.cfm?id=birth-control-in-water-supply

CHAPTER 4

1. I. B. Grafova et al., "Neighborhoods and Obesity in Later Life," *American Journal of Public Health* 98, no. 11 (November 2008): 2065–71.

2. "Sprawl," Merriam-Webster.com, accessed March 13, 2013, http://www.merriam-webster.com/dictionary/sprawl.

3. R. Lopez, "Urban Sprawl and Risk for Being Overweight or Obese," *American Journal of Public Health* 94, no. 9 (September 2004): 1574–79.

4. H. Frumkin, "Urban Sprawl and Public Health," *Public Health Reports* 117, no. 3 (May–June 2002): 201–17.

5. "General Motors Streetcar Conspiracy," *Wikipedia*, last modified September 21, 2013, accessed March 2, 2011, http://en.wikipedia.org/wiki/Great_American_streetcar_scandal.

6. U.S. Census Bureau, "Means of Transportation to Work by Selected Characteristics: 2012 American Community Survey 1-Year Estimates," http://factfinder2.census.gov/faces/tableservices/jsf/pages/productview.xhtml?pid=ACS_12_1YR_S0802&prodType=table.

7. "Palmdale, California," *Wikipedia*, last modified September 24, 2013, accessed March 12, 2013, http://en.wikipedia.org/wiki/Palmdale,_California.

8. Lopez, "Urban Sprawl and Risk for Being Overweight or Obese."

9. Ibid.

10. R. Ewing, R. C. Brownson, and D. Berrigan, "Relationship between Urban Sprawl and Weight of United States Youth," *American Journal of Preventive Medicine* 31, no. 6 (December 2006): 464–74.

11. R. Ewing et al., "Relationship between Urban Sprawl and Physical Activity, Obesity, and Morbidity," *American Journal of Health Promotion* 18, no. 1 (2003): 47–57.

12. Lopez, "Urban Sprawl and Risk for Being Overweight or Obese."

13. Ewing et al., "Relationship between Urban Sprawl and Physical Activity, Obesity, and Morbidity."

14. R. Jackson and C. Kochtitzky, "Creating a Healthy Environment: The Impact of the Built Environment on Public Health" (Washington DC: Sprawl Watch Clearinghouse, 2002).

15. L. Fuzhong et al., "Built Environment, Adiposity, and Physical Activity in Adults Aged 50–75," *American Journal of Preventive Medicine* 36, no. 1 (July 2008): 38–46.

16. Z. Zhao and R. Kaestner, "Effects of Urban Sprawl on Obesity," *Journal of Health Economics* 29, no. 6 (December 2010): 779–87.

17. F. L. Garden and B. B. Jalaludin, "Impact of Urban Sprawl on Overweight, Obesity, and Physical Activity in Sydney, Australia," *Journal of Urban Health* 86, no. 1 (January 2009):19–30.

18. Lopez, "Urban Sprawl and Risk for Being Overweight or Obese."

19. K. Morland, S. Wing, and A. Diez Roux, "The Contextual Effect of the Local Food Environment on Residents' Diets: The Atherosclerosis Risk in Communities Study," *American Journal of Public Health* 92, no. 11 (November 2002): 1761–67.

20. R. W. Jeffery et al., "Are Fast Food Restaurants an Environmental Risk

Factor for Obesity?" *International Journal of Behavioral Nutrition and Physical Activity* 25, no. 3 (January 2006): 2.

21. Lopez, "Urban Sprawl and Risk for Being Overweight or Obese."

22. Ewing et al., "Relationship between Urban Sprawl and Physical Activity, Obesity, and Morbidity."

23. Lopez, "Urban Sprawl and Risk for Being Overweight or Obese."

24. Ibid.

25. R. Ewing, R. Pendall, and D. Chen, "Measuring Sprawl and Its Impact" (Washington, DC: Smart Growth America, 2002).

26. I. M. Lee, R. Ewing, and H. D. Sesso, "The Built Environment and Physical Activity Levels: The Harvard Alumni Health Study," *American Journal of Preventive Medicine* 37, no. 4 (October 2009): 293–98.

27. B. E. Saelens, J. F. Sallis, L. D. Frank, "Environmental Correlates of Walking and Cycling: Findings from the Transportation, Urban Design, and Planning Literatures," *Annals of Behavioral Medicine* 25, no. 2 (Spring 2003): 80–91.

28. L. D. Frank et al., "Stepping Towards Causation: Do Built Environments or Neighborhood and Travel Preferences Explain Physical Activity, Driving, and Obesity?" *Social Science & Medicine* 65, no. 9 (November 2007): 1898–914.

29. A. C. Bell, K. Ge, B. M. Popkin, "The Road to Obesity or the Path to Prevention: Motorized Transportation and Obesity in China," *Obesity Research* 10, no. 4 (April 2002): 277–83.

30. R. Ewing, R. C. Brownson, and D. Berrigan, "Relationship between Urban Sprawl and Weight of United States Youth," *American Journal of Preventive Medicine* 31, no. 6 (December 2006): 464–74.

31. A. J. Plantinga and S. Bernell, "The Association between Urban Sprawl and Obesity: Is It a Two-Way Street?" *Journal of Regional Science* 47, no. 5 (December 2007): 857–79.

32. N. Humpel, N. Owen, and E. Leslie, "Environmental Factors Associated with Adults' Participation in Physical Activity: A Review," *American Journal of Preventive Medicine* 22, no. 3 (April 2002): 188–99.

33. F. L. Garden and B. B. Jalaludin, "Impact of Urban Sprawl on Overweight, Obesity, and Physical Activity in Sydney, Australia," *Journal of Urban Health* 86, no. 1 (January 2009): 19–30.

34. Lopez, "Urban Sprawl and Risk for Being Overweight or Obese."

35. Ewing et al., "Relationship between Urban Sprawl and Physical Activity, Obesity, and Morbidity."

36. J. D. Boardman et al., "Race Differentials in Obesity: The Impact of Place," *Journal of Health and Social Behavior* 46, no. 3 (September 2005): 229–43.

37. S. A. Robert and E. N. Reither, "A Multilevel Analysis of Race, Community Disadvantage, and Body Mass Index among Adults in the US," *Social Science & Medicine* 59, no. 12 (December 2004): 2421–34.

38. I. B. Grafova et al., "Neighborhoods and Obesity in Later Life,"

American Journal of Public Health 98, no. 11 (November 2008): 2065–71

39. A. O. Ferdinand et al., "The Relationship between Built Environments and Physical Activity: A Systematic Review," *American Journal of Public Health* 102, no. 10 (October 2012): e7–e13. doi: 10.2105/AJPH.2012.300740.

40. Leigh Gallagher, *The End of the Suburbs: Where the American Dream Is Moving* (New York: Penguin Group, 2013).

41. "Why Smart Growth?" Smart Growth Online, www.smartgrowth.org/why.php.

42. "This Is Smart Growth," Smart Growth Network (2006), epa.gov/smartgrowth/pdf/2009_11_tisg.pdf.

43. Centers for Disease Control, "Progress on Childhood Obesity," accessed August 2013, http://www.cdc.gov/vitalsigns/childhoodobesity.

44. Centers for Disease Control and Prevention, "The Guide to Community Preventive Services: Tobacco Use and Prevention," *American Journal of Preventive Medicine* 20, suppl. (2001): 1–88.

45. L. D. Frank et al., "Linking Objectively Measured Physical Activity with Objectively Measured Urban Form: Findings from SMARTRAQ," *American Journal of Preventive Medicine* 28, no. 2, suppl. 2 (February 2005): 117–25.

46. Berke EM et al., "Association of the Built Environment with Physical Activity and Obesity in Older Persons," *American Journal of Public Health* 97, no. 3 (March 2007)): 486–92. doi:10.2105/AJPH.2006.

47. Lee, Ewing, and Sesso, "The Built Environment and Physical Activity Levels."

48. Frumkin, "Urban Sprawl and Public Health."

49. "History of the Bicycle," Wikipedia, accessed March 2, 2011, http://en.wikipedia.org/wiki/History_of_the_bicycle.

50. "Road Traffic Injuries Fact Sheet," World Health Organization, http://www.who.int/mediacentre/factsheets/fs358/en.

CHAPTER 5

1. Tina Susman, "Another Iraqi Casualty of War: Their Waistlines," *Los Angeles Times*, Sept. 8, 2008, http://articles.latimes.com/2008/sep/08/world/fg-fat8.

2. H. L. Burdette, T. A. Wadden, and R. C. Whitaker, "Neighborhood Safety, Collective Efficacy, and Obesity in Women with Young Children," *Obesity* 14 (2006): 518–25.

3. N. Pecoraro et al., "Chronic Stress Promotes Palatable Feeding, Which Reduces Signs of Stress: Feedforward and Feedback Effects of Chronic Stress," *Endocrinology* 145, no. 8 (August 2004): 3754–62.

4. L. A. Weir, D. Etelson, and D. A. Brand, "Parents' Perceptions of Neighborhood Safety and Children's Physical Activity," *Preventive Medicine* 43, no. 3 (September 2006): 212–17.

5. T. K. Boehmer et al., "What Constitutes an Obesogenic Environment in Rural Communities?" *American Journal of Health Promotion* 20, no. 6 (July–August 2006): 411–21.

6. J. E. Gómez et al., "Violent Crime and Outdoor Physical Activity among Inner-City Youth," *Preventive Medicine* 39, no. 5 (November 2004): 876–81.

7. H. S. Brown et al., "Crime Rates and Sedentary Behavior among 4th Grade Texas School Children," *International Journal of Behavioral Nutrition and Physical Activity* 5 (2008): 28.

8. Ibid.

9. Ibid.

10. J. B. Moore et al., "A Qualitative Examination of Perceived Barriers and Facilitators of Physical Activity for Urban and Rural Youth," *Health Education Research* 25, no. 2 (April 2010): 355–67.

11. P. Veugelers et al., "Neighborhood Characteristics in Relation to Diet, Physical Activity and Overweight of Canadian Children," *International Journal of Pediatric Obesity* 3, no. 3 (2008): 152–59.

12. S. S. Casagrande et al., "Built Environment and Health Behaviors among African Americans: A Systematic Review," *American Journal of Preventive Medicine* 36, no. 2 (February 2009): 174–81.

13. H. L. Burdette and R. C. Whitaker, "Neighborhood Playgrounds, Fast Food Restaurants, and Crime: Relationships to Overweight in Low-Income Preschool Children," *Preventive Medicine* 38, no. 1 (January 2004): 57–63.

14. Gary G. Bennett, Dustin T. Duncan, and Kathleen Y. Wolin, "Social Determinants of Obesity" in Frank B. Hu, ed., *Obesity Epidemiology* (New York, Oxford University Press, 2008), 136.

15. United Nations Statistic Division, "Intentional Homicide, Number and Rate per 100,000 Population, accessed August 18, 2013, http://data.un.org/Data.aspx?d=UNODC&f=tableCode%3A1.

16. N. C. McDonald, "The Effect of Objectively Measured Crime on Walking in Minority Adults," *American Journal of Health Promotion* 22, no. 6 (July–August 2008): 433–36.

17. C. C. Weiss et al., "Reconsidering Access: Park Facilities and Neighborhood Disamenities in New York City," *Journal of Urban Health* 88, no. 11 (April 2011): 297–310.

18. G. S. Lovasi et al., "Built Environments and Obesity in Disadvantaged Populations," *Epidemiologic Reviews* 31, no. 1 (2009): 7–20.

19. D. K. Wilson et al., "An Overview of the "Positive Action for Today's Health" (PATH) Trial for Increasing Walking in Low Income, Ethnic Minority Communities," *Contemporary Clinical Trials* 31, no. 6 (November 2010): 624–33.

20. H. S. Brown et al., "Crime Rates and Sedentary Behavior among 4th Grade Texas School Children," *International Journal of Behavioral Nutrition and Physical Activity* 5 (2008): 28.

21. D. F. Williamson et al., "Body Weight and Obesity in Adults and

Self-Reported Abuse in Childhood," *International Journal of Obesity* 26, no. 8 (August 2002): 1075–82.

22. V. J. Felitti, "Long-Term Medical Consequences of Incest, Rape, and Molestation," *Southern Medical Journal* 84, no. 3 (March 1991): 328–31.

23. T. A. Wadden et al., "Comparison of Psychosocial Status in Treatment-Seeking Women with Class III vs. Class I-II Obesity," *Surgery for Obesity & Related Diseases.* 2006;2:138–45.

24. C. M. Grilo et al., "Childhood Maltreatment in Extremely Obese Male and Female Bariatric Surgery Candidates," *Obesity Research* 13, no. 1 (January 2005): 123–30.

25. J. E. Wildes et al., "Childhood Maltreatment and Psychiatric Morbidity in Bariatric Surgery Candidates," *Obes Surgery* 18, no. 3 (March 2008): 306–13.

26. V. J. Felitti, "Childhood Sexual Abuse, Depression, and Family Dysfunction in Adult Obese Patients: A Case Control Study," *Southern Medical Journal* 86, no. 7 (July 1993): 732–36.

27. C. Thomas, E. Hyppönen, and C. Power, "Obesity and Type 2 Diabetes Risk in Midadult Life: The Role of Childhood Adversity," *Pediatrics* 121, no. 5 (May 2008): e1240–49. doi: 10.1542/peds.2007-2403.

28. A. A. Mamun et al., "Does Childhood Sexual Abuse Predict Young Adult's BMI? A Birth Cohort Study," *Obesity* (Silver Spring, MD) 15, no. 8 (August 2007): 2103–10.

29. O. Pinhas-Hamiel et al., "Obesity in Girls and Penetrative Sexual Abuse in Childhood," *Acta Paediatricia* 98, no. 1 (January 2009): 144–47.

30. J. G. Noll et al., "Obesity Risk for Female Victims of Childhood Sexual Abuse: A Prospective Study," *Pediatrics* 120, no. 1 (July 2007): e61–67.

31. P. Rohde et al., "Associations of Child Sexual and Physical Abuse with Obesity and Depression in Middle-Aged Women," *Child Abuse & Neglect Journal* 32, no. 9 (September 2008): 878–87.

32. Hee-Jin et al., "Growing Up in a Domestic Violence Environment: Relationship with Developmental Trajectories of Body Mass Index during Adolescence into Young Adulthood," *Journal of Epidemiology & Community Health* 66 (2012): 629–35. doi:10.1136/jech.2010.110932.

33. R. C. Whitaker et al., "The Association between Maltreatment and Obesity among Preschool Children," *Child Abuse & Neglect Journal* 31, nos. 11–12 (November–December 2007): 1187–99.

34. Felitti, "Childhood Sexual Abuse, Depression, and Family Dysfunction."

35. E. A. Greenfield and N. F. Marks, "Violence from Parents in Childhood and Obesity in Adulthood: Using Food in Response to Stress As a Mediator of Risk," *Social Science & Medicine* 68, no. 5 (March 2009): 791–98.

36. E. McCrory, S. S. De Brito, and E. Viding, "The Impact of Childhood Maltreatment: A Review of Neurobiological and Genetic Factors," *Frontiers in Psychiatry* 2 (2011): 48.

37. A. J. Midei, K. A. Matthews, and Joyce T. Bromberger, "Childhood

Abuse is Associated with Adiposity in Mid-life Women: Possible Pathways through Trait Anger and Reproductive Hormones," *Psychosomatic Medicine* 72, no. 2 (February 2010): 215–23.

38. K. Räikkönen, K. A. Matthews, and L. H. Kuller, "Anthropometric and Psychosocial Determinants of Visceral Obesity in Healthy Postmenopausal Women," *International Journal of Obesity* 23, no. 8 (August 1999): 775–82.

39. A. J. Midei and K. A. Matthews, "Social Relationships and Negative Emotional Traits Are Associated with Central Adiposity and Arterial Stiffness in Healthy Adolescents," *Health Psychology Journal* 28, no. 3 (May 2009): 347–53.

40. Midei, Matthews, and Bromberger, "Childhood Abuse Is Associated with Adiposity in Mid-life Women."

41. T. B. Gustafson and D. B. Sarwer, "Childhood Sexual Abuse and Obesity," *Obesity Reviews* 5, no. 3 (August 2004): 129–35.

42. E. A. Greenfield and N. F. Marks, "Violence from Parents in Childhood and Obesity in Adulthood: Using Food in Response to Stress as a Mediator of Risk," *Social Science & Medicine* 68, no. 5 (March 2009): 791–98.

43. Whitaker et al., "The Association between Maltreatment and Obesity among Preschool Children."

CHAPTER 6

1. Global Health Report on Non-communicable Diseases. World Health Organization, 2010.

2. B. A. Swinburn et al., "The Global Obesity Pandemic: Shaped by Global Drivers and Local Environments," *Lancet* 378, no. 9793 (August 27, 2011): 804–14. doi: 10.1016/S0140-6736(11)60813-1.

3. Ibid.

4. Marion Nestle, *Food Politics: How the Food Industry Influences Nutrition and Health* (Los Angeles: University of California Press, 2003).

5. Ibid.

6. Ibid.

7. R. G. Wilkinson and K. E. Pickett, "Income Inequality and Population Health: A Review and Explanation of the Evidence," *Social Science & Medicine* 62, no. 7 (April 2006): 1768–84.

8. J. F. Guthrie, B. H. Lin, and E. Frazao, "Role of Food Prepared Away from Home in the American Diet, 1977–78 versus 1994–96: Changes and Consequences," *Journal of Nutrition and Education Behavior* 34, no. 3 (May–June 2002): 140–50.

9. US Department of Agriculture, Economic Research Service Food CPI, "Prices and Expenditures: Foodservice As a Share of Food Expenditures, a, http://www.ers.usda.gov/Briefing?CPIFoodAndExpenditures/Data/table12.htm.

10. R. R. Briefel and C. L. Johnson CL, "Secular Trends in Dietary Intake in the United States," *Annual Review of Nutrition* 24 (2004): 401–31.

11. Nestle, *Food Politics*.

12. B. Anderson et al., "Fast-Food Consumption and Obesity among Michigan Adults," *Preventing Chronic Disease* 8, no. 4 (July 2011): A71.

13. Jason Straziuso, "KFC Goes to Kenya; First U.S. Fast-Food Chain in E. Africa," Associated Press, for *USA TODAY*, August 23, 2011, http://usatoday30.usatoday.com/money/industries/food/story/2011-08-27/KFC-goes-to-Kenya-first-US-fast-food-chain-in-E-Africa/50108550/1.

14. N. P. Steyn, D. Labadarios, and J. H. Nel, "Factors Which Influence the Consumption of Street Foods and Fast Foods in South Africa—A National Survey," *Nutrition Journal* 10, no. 1 (October 2011): 104.

15. Morgan Spurlock, *Don't Eat This Book: Fast Food and the Supersizing of America* (New York: G. P. Putnam's Sons, 2005).

16. S. A. Bowman, B. T. Vinyard, "Fast Food Consumption of US Adults: Impact on Energy and Nutrient Intakes and Overweight Status," *Journal of the American College of Nutrition* 23, no. 2 (April 2004): 163–68.

17. B. Anderson et al., "Fast-Food Consumption and Obesity among Michigan Adults," *Preventing Chronic Disease* 8, no. 4 (July 2011): A71.

18. S. E. Fleischhacker et al., "A Systematic Review of Fast Food Access Studies," *Obesity Reviews* 12, no. 5 (2011).

19. A. S. Richardson et al., "Neighborhood Fast Food Restaurants and Fast Food Consumption: A National Study," *BMC Public Health* 11 (July 8, 2011: 543.

20. Tom Vanderbilt, "We're Thru," *Slate Magazine*, December 11, 2009.

21. April Dembosky, "KFC Eyes More Orders with 'Mobile Wallet'," *Financial Times,* April 3, 2013, 22.

22. A. K. Garber and R. H. Lustig, "Is Fast Food Addictive?" *Current Drug Abuse Reviews*, September 1, 2011.

23. Barbara Rolls and Robert A. Barnett, *The Volumetrics Weight-Control Plan* (New York: HarperTorch, 2002)

24. Lorie Parch, "The Secrets of Thin People," *Real Simple* online, accessed March 26, 2013, http://www.realsimple.com/health/nutrition-diet/weight-loss/secrets-thin-people-10000001170137/print-index.html.

25. H. Stewart, N. Blisard, and D. Jolliffen "Let's Eat Out: Americans Weigh Taste, Convenience, and Nutrition," *Economic Information Bulletin*, no. EIB-19, October 2006, http://www.ers.usda.gov/publications/eib19/eib19.pdf

26. Morgan Spurlock, *Don't Eat This Book: Fast Food and the Supersizing of America* (New York: G.P. Putnam's Sons, 2005).

27. N. I. Larson, M. T. Story, M. C. Nelson, "Neighborhood Environments: Disparities in Access to Healthy Foods in the U.S," *American Journal of Preventive Medicine* 36, no. 1 (January 2009): 74–81.

28. "Food Environment Atlas: Overview," Economic Research Service, United States Department of Agriculture, last modified September 18, 2013, http://www.ers.usda.gov/data-products/food-environment-atlas.aspx.

29. Ploeq et. al, "Access to Affordable and Nutritious Food—Measuring

and Understanding Food Deserts and Their Consequences: Report to Congress," USDA, June 2009.

30. H. Lee, "The Role of Local Food Availability in Explaining Obesity Risk among Young School-Aged Children," *Social Science & Medicine* 74, no. 8 (April 2012)): 1193–203. doi: 10.1016/j.socscimed.2011.12.036.

31. Ploeq et. al, "Access to Affordable and Nutritious Food."

32. J. Boone-Heinonen et al., "Fast Food Restaurants and Food Stores: Longitudinal Associations with Diet in Young to Middle-Aged Adults: The CARDIA Study," *Archives of Internal Medicine* 171, no. 13 (July 11, 2011): 1162–70.

33. Ruopeng An and R. Sturm, "School and Residential Neighborhood Food Environment and Diet among California Youth," *American Journal of Preventive Medicine* 42, no. 2 (February 1, 2012): 129–35.

34. T. Hanibuchi et al., "Neighborhood Food Environment and Body Mass Index among Japanese Older Adults: Results from the Aichi Gerontological Evaluation Study (AGES)," *International Journal of Health Geographics* 10, no. 1 (July 21, 2011): 43.

35. S. L. Gortmaker et al., "Changing the Future of Obesity: Science, Policy, and Action," *Lancet* 378, no. 9793 (August 27, 2011): 838–47

36. C. Courtemanche and A. Carden, "Supersizing Supercenters? The Impact of Wal-Mart Supercenters on Body Mass Index and Obesity," September 10, 2010, http://ssrn.com/abstract=1263316 or http://dx.doi.org/10.2139/ssrn.1263316

37. Greg Critser, *Fat Land* (New York: Penguin Books, 2003).

38. P. H. Howard, M. Fitzpatrick, and B. Fulfrost, "Proximity of Food Retailers to Schools and Rates of Overweight Ninth Grade Students: An Ecological Study in California," *BMC Public Health* 11 (January 31, 2011): 68.

39. Julie Jargon, "How Lunchtime is Turning into Snack Time," *Wall Street Journal,* September 8, 2010.

40. R. Sebastian et al., "Snacking Patterns in U.S. Adults: What We Eat in America, NHANES 2007–2008," *Food Surveys Research GroupDietary Data Brief,* no. 4 (June 2011), http://ars.usda.gov/SP2UserFiles/Place/12355000/pdf/DBrief/4_adult_snacking_0708.pdf

41. C. Piernas and B. M. Popkin, "Trends in Snacking among U.S. Children," *Health Affairs* (Millwood, MD) 29, no. 3 (March–April 2010): 398–404.

42. "Fourthmeal," UrbanDictionary.com, http://www.urbandictionary.com/define.php?term=fourthmeal.

43. Critser, *Fat Land.*

44. E. L. Morris et al., "Portion Size of Food Influences Energy Intake in Adults," *FASEB Journal* 15 (March 8, 2001): A890.

45. "Nearly Half of Americans Drink Soday Daily," *Gallup Wellbeing,* http://www.gallup.com/poll/156116/Nearly-Half-Americans-Drink-Soda-Daily.aspx.

46. R. J. Johnson et al., "Potential Role of Sugar (Fructose) in the Epidemic

of Hypertension, Obesity and the Metabolic Syndrome, Diabetes, Kidney Disease, and Cardiovascular Disease," *American Journal of Clinical Nutrition* 86, no. 4 (October 2007): 899–906.

47.   Q. Shao and K. V. Chin, "Survey of American Food Trends and the Growing Obesity Epidemic," *Nutrition Research and Practice*. 2011 Jun;5(3):253–9.

48.   Duane Stanford, "Africa: Coke's Last Frontier," *BusinessWeek*, October 28, 2010.

49.   "International Year of the Potato," FAO, accessed November 21, 2011, http://www.potato2008.org/en/world/northamerica.html.

50.   D. Mozaffarian et al., "Changes in diet and lifestyle and long-term weight gain in women and men," New England Journal of Medicine. 364, no. 5 (June 23, 2011): 2392–404

51.   "SNAP/Foodstamp Participation," Food Research and Action Center, http://frac.org/reports-and-resources/snapfood-stamp-monthly-participation-data.

52.   "Supplemental Nutrition Assistance Program: Eligibility," USDA Food and Nutrition Service, last modified September 30, 2013, http://www.fns.usda.gov/snap/applicant_recipients/eligibility.htm

53.   J. D. Shenkin and M. F. Jacobson MF, "Using the Food Stamp Program and Other Methods to Promote Healthy Diets for Low-Income Consumers," *American Journal of Public Health* 100, no. 9 (September 2010): 1562–64.

54.   Patrick McGeehan, "Federal Officials Reject City's Plan to Ban Food Stamps for Soda," *New York Times,* August 19, 2011, http://cityroom. blogs.nytimes.com/2011/08/19/washington-rejects-n-y-c-ban-on-use-of-food-stamps-to-buy-sodas/

55.   "Supplemental Nutrition Assistance Program: Eligible Food Items," USDA Food and Nutrition Service, last modified November 5, 2013, http://ww.fns.usda.gov/snap/retailers/eligible.htm

56.   Eric A. Finkelstein and Laurie Zuckerman, *The Fattening of America* (Hoboken, NJ: John Wiley & Sons, 2008), p. 126

57.   Mark Bittman, "Is Junk Food Really Cheaper?" *New York Times*, September 24, 2011.

58.   Lucia A. Reisch et al., "Experimental Evidence on the Impact of Food Advertising on Children's Knowledge about and Preferences for Healthful Food," *Journal of Obesity* vol. 2013 (2013), Article ID 408582. doi:10.1155/2013/408582.

59.   Michael Pollan, *In Defense of Food: An Eater's Manifesto* (New York: Penguin Books, 2009), p. 1.

60.   Eric Schlosser, *Fast Food Nation* (New York: Penguin Putnam, 2001).

61.   Christina A. Roberto, et al., "Influence of Licensed Characters on Children's Taste and Snack Preferences," *Pediatrics* 126, no. 1 (July 1, 2010): 88–93.

62.   T. N. Robinson, et al., "The Effects of Fast Food Branding on Young Children's Taste Preferences," *Archives of Pediatrics & Adolescent Medicine* 161, no. 8 (August 2007): 792–97.

63. S. Linn and C. L. Novosat, "Calories for Sale: Food Marketing to Children in the Twenty-First Century," *Annals of the American Academy of Political and Social Science* 615, no. 1 (January 2008): 133–55

64. C. A. Roberto et al., "Influence of Licensed Characters on Children's Taste and Snack Preferences," *Pediatrics* 126, no. 1 (July 2010): 88–93.

65. A. S. Levy and R. C. Stokes, " Effects of a Health Promotion Advertising Campaign on Sales of Ready-To-Eat Cereals," *Public Health Reports* 102, no. 4 (July–August 1987): 398–403.

66. "10 Strange, Bizarre, and Unusual Restaurants," *Daily Fork*, accessed August 8, 2013, http://www.dailyfork.com/2009/05/10_strange_bizarre_and _unusual.php?page=2.

67. "Competitive Eating," *Wikipedia*, accessed March 28, 2013, http:// en.wikipedia.org/wiki/Competitive_eating.

68. "Hara hachi bu," Wikipedia, accessed March 28, 2013, http:// en.wikipedia.org/wiki/Hara_hachi_bu.

69. M. Chan, "Noncommunicable Diseases Damage Health, Including Economic Health," address at the High-Level Meeting on Noncommunicable Diseases, United Nations General Assembly, New York, September 19, 2011.

70. B. A. Swinburn et al., "The Global Obesity Pandemic: Shaped by Global Drivers and Local Environments," *Lancet* 378, no. 9793 (August 27, 2011): 804–14. doi: 10.1016/S0140-6736(11)60813-1.

71. K. D. Brownell and T. R. Frieden, "Ounces of Prevention—The Public Policy Case for Taxes on Sugared Beverages," *New England Journal of Medicine* 360, no. 18 (April 30, 2009): 1805–8.

72. D. R. Taber et al., "Banning All Sugar-Sweetened Beverages in Middle Schools: Reduction of In-School Access and Purchasing but Not Overall Consumption," *Archives of Pediatrics & Adolescent Medicine* 166, no. 3 (March 2012): 256–62. doi: 10.1001/archpediatrics.2011.200.

73. Suzanne Daley, "Hungary Tries a Dash of Taxes to Promote Healthier Eating Habits," *New York Times*, March 3, 2013, www.nytimes.com/2013/03/03 /world/europe/hungary-experiments-with-food-tax-to-coax-healthier-habits. html.

74. A. Asfaw, "Do Government Food Price Policies Affect the Prevalence of Obesity? Empirical Evidence from Egypt," *World Development* 35, no. 4 (April 2007): 687–701

75. USDA, "Healthy Incentives Pilot (HIP) Interim Report—Summary," July 2013, accessed November 18, 2011, http://www.fns.usda.gov/ORA/menu/ Published/SNAP/FILES/ProgramDesign/HIP_Interim_Summary. pdf.

76. A. M. Thow, S. Jan, S. Leeder, B. Swinburn. "The Effect of Fiscal Policy on Diet, Obesity and Chronic Disease: A Systematic Review," *Bulletin of the World Health Organization* 88, no. 8 (August 1, 2010): 609–614. doi: 10.2471/ BLT.2409.070987.

77. L. M. Powell and F. J. Chaloupka, "Food Prices and Obesity: Evidence

and Policy Implications for Taxes and Subsidies," *Milbank Quarterly* 87, no. 1 (March 2009): 229–57. doi: 10.1111/j.1468-0009.2009.00554.x.

78. H. Eyles et al., "Food Pricing Strategies, Population Diets, and Non-Communicable Disease: A Systematic Review of Simulation Studies," *Public Library of Science Medicine* 9, no. 12 (December 2012): e1001353. doi: 10.1371/journal.pmed.1001353

79. Claudia Chaufan, et al., "Taxing 'Sin Foods'—Obesity Prevention and Public Health Policy," *New England Journal of Medicine* 61 (December 10, 2009): e113.

80. Suzanne Daley, "Hungary Tries a Dash of Taxes to Promote Healthier Eating Habits," *New York Times*, March 2, 2013.

81. David Bornstein, "Conquering Food Deserts with Green Carts," *New York Times*, April 18, 2012, http://opinionator.blogs.nytimes.com/2012/04/18/conquering-food-deserts-with-green-carts/ Accessed March 28, 2013

82. "Philadelphia's Healthy Corner Store Initiative: 2010-2012 Report," accessed March 28, 2013, http://foodtrust-prod.punkave.net/uploads/media_items/hcsi-y2report-final.original.pdf.

83. Morgan Spurlock, *Super Size Me* (Snagfilms, 2012).

84. S. Bernstein, "Restaurants to Offer More-Healthful Fare for Kids," *Los Angeles Times*, July 13, 2011, articles.latimes.com/2011/jul/13/business/la-fi-restaurants-kids-20110713.

85. "'Better for You' Foods Also Better for Profits," News Bite, Tufts University Health and Nutrition Letter, January 2012, www.tuftshealthletter.com/showArticle.aspx?RowID=1060.

86. B. Elbel, J. Gyamfi, and R. Kersh, "Child and Adolescent Fast-Food Choice and the Influence of Calorie Labeling: A Natural Experiment," *International Journal of Obesity* 35, no. 4 (April 2011): 493–500. doi:10.1038/ijo.2011.4.

87. C. A. Roberto et al., "Evaluating the Impact of Menu Labeling on Food Choices and Intake," *American Journal of Public Health* 100, no. 3 (February 2010): 312–18.

88. B. Anderson et al., "Fast-Food Consumption and Obesity among Michigan Adults," *Preventing Chronic Disease* 8, no. 4 (July 2011): A71.

89. S. D. Sugarman and N. Sandman, "Using Performance-Based Regulation to Reduce Childhood Obesity," *Australia and New Zealand Health Policy* 5 (November 18, 2008): 26.

90. M. M. Slining, S. W. Ng, and B. M. Popkin, "Food Companies' Calorie-Reduction Pledges to Improve U.S. Diet," *American Journal of Preventive Medicine* 44, no. 2 (February 2013): 174–84. doi: 10.1016/j.amepre.2012.09.064.

91. "Global Dump Soft Drinks Campaign," accessed March 28, 2013, http://www.dumpsoda.org.

92. "Disney to Banish Junk-Food Ads from Kid Shows," Staff Report, *New York Post*, June 5, 2012, disney-to-banish-junk-food-ads-from-kid-shows.

93. Anahad O'Connor, "Bans on School Junk Food Pay Off in California,"

New York Times, May 8, 2012, http://well.blogs.nytimes.com/2012/05/08/bans-on-school-junk-food-pay-off-in-california.

94. "CED Data: Healthy Food Financing Initiative," Administration for Children & Families, January 18, 2011, http://www.acf.hhs.gov/programs/ocs/resource/healthy-food-financing-initiative-0.

95. "Restaurants to Offer More-Healthful Fare for Kids," *Los Angeles Times*, July 12, 2011, http://articles.latimes.com/2011/jul/13/business/la-fi-restaurants-kids-20110713.

96. M. Grynbaum, "New York Soda Ban to Go Before State's Top Court," *New York Times*, October 17, 2013, http://www.nytimes.com/2013/10/18/nyregion/new-york-soda-ban-to-go-before-states-top-court.html?_r=0.

CHAPTER 7

1. R. J. Schilder and J. H. Marden, "Metabolic Syndrome and Obesity in an Insect," *Proceedings of the National Academy of Sciences of the United States of America* 103, no. 49 (December 5, 2006):18805–9.

2. R. L. Atkinson et al., "Human Adenovirus-36 Is Associated with Increased Body Weight and Paradoxical Reduction of Serum Lipids," *International Journal of Obesity* (London) 29, no. 3 (March 2005): 286–87.

3. Maggie Fox, "U.S. Apologizes for Syphilis Study in Guatemala," *Reuters*, October 1, 2010, accessed January 18, 2011, http://www.reuters.com/article/2010/10/01/us-usa-guatemala-experiment-idUSTRE6903RZ20101001.

4. Atkinson et al., "Human Adenovirus-36."

5. C. Gabbert, et al., "Adenovirus 36 and Obesity in Children and Adolescents," *Pediatrics* 126, no. 4 (October 2010): 721–26

6. L. D. Whigham, B. A. Israel, and R. L. Atkinson, "Adipogenic Potential of Multiple Human Adenoviruses In Vivo and In Vitro in Animals," *American Journal of Physiology - Regulatory, Integrative and Comparative Physiology* 290, no. 1 (January 2006): R190–94.

7. Atkinson et al., "Human Adenovirus-36."

8. T. Yamada, K. Hara, and T. Kadowaki, "Association of Adenovirus 36 Infection with Obesity and Metabolic Markers in Humans: A Meta-Analysis of Observational Studies," *PLOS ONE* 7, no. 7 (July 2012): e42031. doi: 10.1371/journal.pone.0042031.

9. E. J. McAllister et al., "Ten Putative Contributors to the Obesity Epidemic," *Critical Reviews in Food Science & Nutrition* 49, no. 10 (November 2009): 868–913.

10. R. L. Atkinson, "Viruses As an Etiology of Obesity," *Mayo Clinic Proceedings* 82, no. 10 (October 2007): 1192–98.

11. McAllister et al., "Ten Putative Contributors to the Obesity Epidemic."

12. N. V. Dhurandhar, "A Framework for Identification of Infections That Contribute to Human Obesity," *Lancet Infectious Diseases* 11, no 12 (December 2011): 963–69.

13. Ibid.

14. N. V. Dhurandhar, "Infectobesity: Obesity of Infectious Origin," *Journal of Nutrition* 131, no. 10 (October 2001): 2794S–97S.

15. V. Hegde and N. V. Dhurandhar, "Microbes and Obesity—Interrelationship between Infection, Adipose Tissue and the Immune System," *Clinical Microbiology and Infections* 19, no. 4 (April 2013): 314–20.

16. E. Isolauri, "Development of Healthy Gut Microbiota Early in Life," *Journal of Paediatrics and Child Health* 48, suppl. 3 (June 2012): 1–6.

17. Rachel Browne, "C-Section Babies at Higher Risk of Obesity," *BrisbaneTimes.com.au*, March 18, 2012, http://www.brisbanetimes.com.au/national /health/csection-babies-at-higher-risk-of-obesity-20120317-1vc22.html

18. J. A. Martin et al., "Births: Final Data for 2011," *National Vital Statistics Reports* 62, no. 1 (June 2013), accessed March 30, 2013, http://www.cdc.gov/nchs /fastats/delivery.htm.

19. L. Gibbons et al., "The Global Numbers and Costs of Additionally Needed and Unnecessary Cesarean Sections Performed per Year: Overuse as a Barrier to Universal Coverage," World Health Organization, 2010, http://www. who.int/healthsystems/topics/financing/healthreport/30C-sectioncosts.pdf.

20. S. Y. Huh et al., "Delivery by Cesarean Section and Risk of Obesity in Preschool Age Children: A Prospective Cohort Study," *Archives of Disease in Childhood* 97, no. 7 (July 2012): 610–16. doi: 10.1136/archdischild-2011-301141.

21. R. Luoto et al., "Initial Dietary and Microbiological Environments Deviation in Normal-Weight Compared to Overweight Children at 10 Years of Age," *Journal of Pediatric Gastroenterology and Nutrition* 52, no. 1 (January 2011): 90–95.

22. F. Bäckhed, "99th Dahlem Conference on Infection, Inflammation and Chronic Inflammatory Disorders: The Normal Gut Microbiota in Health and Disease," *Clinical and Experimental Immunology* 160, no 1 (April 2010): 80–4. doi: 10.1111/j.1365-2249.2010.04123.x.

23. "Making Health Care Safer: Stopping C. difficile Infections," Centers for Disease Control and Prevention, *VitalSigns* (March 2012), http://www.cdc .gov/VitalSigns/Hai/StoppingCdifficile.

24. "Microbes," National Institute of Allergy and Infectious Diseases, last modified April 3, 2012, http://www.niaid.nih.gov/topics/microbes/PAges/default .aspx.

25. Bäckhed, "The Normal Gut Microbiota in Health and Disease."

26. F. Bäckhed et al., "The Gut Microbiota As an Environmental Factor That Regulates Fat Storage," *Proceedings of the National Academy of Sciences of the United States of America* 101, no. 44 (November 2004): 15718–23.."

27. R. E. Ley et al., "Microbial Ecology: Human Gut Microbes Associated with Obesity," *Nature* 444, no. 7122 (December 2006): 1022–23

28. Bäckhed, "The Normal Gut Microbiota in Health and Disease."

29. Bäckhed et al., "The Gut Microbiota As an Environmental Factor That Regulates Fat Storage."

30. F. Bäckhed et al., "Mechanisms Underlying the Resistance to Diet-Induced Obesity in Germ-Free Mice," *Proceedings of the National Academy of Sciences of the United States of America* 104, no. 3 (January 16, 2007): 979–84.

31. P. J. Turnbaugh et al., "The Effect of Diet on the Human Gut Microbiome: A Metagenomic Analysis in Humanized Gnotobiotic Mice," *Science Translational Medicine* 1, no. 6 (November 11, 2009): 6ra14.

32. P. J. Turnbaugh et al., "An Obesity-Associated Gut Microbiome with Increased Capacity for Energy Harvest," *Nature* 444, no. 7122 (December 21, 2006): 1027–31.

33. Ibid.

34. R. E. Ley et al., "Microbial Ecology: Human Gut Microbes Associated with Obesity," *Nature* 444, no. 7122 (December 2006): 1022–23.

35. C. De Filippo et al., "Impact of Diet in Shaping Gut Microbiota Revealed by a Comparative Study in Children from Europe and Rural Africa," *Proceedings of the National Academy of Sciences of the United States of America* 107, no. 33 (August 17, 2010):14691–96.

36. J. H. Kang, S. I. Yun, and H. O. Park, "Effects of Lactobacillus Gasseri BNR17 on Body Weight and Adipose Tissue Mass in Diet-Induced Overweight Rats," *Journal of Microbiology* 48, no. 5 (October 2010): 712–14.

37. L. Aronsson, et al., "Decreased Fat Storage by *Lactobacillus paracasei* Is Associated with Increased Levels of Angiopoietin-Like 4 Protein (ANGPTL4)," *PLOS ONE* 5, no. 9 (September 30, 2010), doi: 10.1371/journal.pone.001387.

38. N. Takemura, T. Okubo, and K. Sonoyama, "*Lactobacillus plantarum* Strain No. 14 Reduces Adipocyte Size in Mice Fed High-Fat Diet," *Experimental Biology and Medicine* (Maywood, NJ) 235, no. 7 (July 2010): 849–56.

39. M. Million, et al., "Obesity-Associated Gut Microbiota Is Enriched in Lactobacillus Reuteri and Depleted in *Bifidobacterium animalis* and *Methanobrevibacter smithii*," *International Journal of Obesity* (London) 36, no. 6 (June 2012): 817–25

40. M. Khan, et al., "Growth-Promoting Effects of Single-Dose Intragastrically Administered Probiotics in Chickens," *British Poultry Science* 48, no. 6 (December 2007): 732–35.

41. N. Vendt, et al., "Growth during the First 6 Months of Life in Infants Using Formula Enriched with *Lactobacillus rhamnosus* GG: Double-Blind, Randomized Trial," *Journal of Human Nutrition and Dietetics* 19, no. 1 (February 2006): 51–58.

42. H. M. An et al., "Antiobesity and Lipid-Lowering Effects of Bifidobacterium Spp. in High Fat Diet-Induced Obese Rats," *Lipids in Health and Disease* 10, vol. 116 (July 12, 2011), doi:10.1186/1476-511x-10-116

43. S. D. Feighner and M. P. Dashkevicz, "Subtherapeutic Levels of Antibiotics in Poultry Feeds and Their Effects on Weight Gain, Feed Efficiency, and Bacterial Cholyltaurine Hydrolase Activity," *Applied Environmental Microbiology* 53, no. 2 (February 1987): 331–36.

44. F. Thuny et al., "Vancomycin Treatment of Infective Endocarditis Is Linked with Recently Acquired Obesity," *PLOS ONE* 5, no. 2 (Februar 2010): e9074.

45. L. Trasande et al., "Infant Antibiotic Exposures and Early-Life Body Mass," *International Journal of Obesity* 37 (2013): 16–23. doi:10.1038/ijo.2012.132.

46. L. Dethlefsen et al., "The Pervasive Effects of an Antibiotic on the Human Gut Microbiota, As Revealed by Deep 16S rRNA Sequencing," *PLoS Biology* 6, no. 11 (November 18, 2008): 2383–2400.

47. J. Penders et al., "Factors Influencing the Composition of the Intestinal Microbiota in Early Infancy," *Pediatrics* 118, no. 2 (August 2006): 511–21.

48. I. H. Rosenberg et al., "Infant and Child Enteritis-Malabsorption-Malnutrition: The Potential of Limited Studies with Low-Dose Antibiotic Feeding," *American Journal of Clinical Nutrition* 27, no. 3 (March 1974): 304–9.

49. N. A. Christakis and J. H. Fowler, "The Spread of Obesity in a Large Social Network Over 32 Years," *New England Journal of Medicine* 357, no. 4 (July 26, 2007: 370–79.

50. T. M. Leahey et al., "Social Influences Are Associated with BMI and Weight Loss Intentions in Young Adults," *Obesity* (Silver Spring, MD) 19, no. 6 (June 2011): 1157–62.

51. McAllister et al., "Ten Putative Contributors to the Obesity Epidemic."

52. A. A. Gorin et al., "Weight Loss Treatment Influences Untreated Spouses and the Home Environment: Evidence of a Ripple Effect," *International Journal of Obesity* 32, no. 11 (November 2008), 1678–84.

53. K. Cline and K. Ferraro, "Does Religion Increase the Prevalence and Incidence of Obesity in Adulthood?" *Journal of the Scientific Study of Religion* 45, no. 2 (June 2006): 269–281.

54. R. Chunara et al., "Assessing the Online Social Environment for Surveillance of Obesity Prevalence," *PLOS ONE* 8, no. 4 (April 24, 2013): e61373. doi: 10.1371/journal.pone.0061373.

55. N. V. Dhurandhar, "A Framework for Identification of Infections."

56. J. Lin, "Effect of Antibiotic Growth Promoters on Intestinal Microbiota in Food Animals: A Novel Model for Studying the Relationship between Gut Microbiota and Human Obesity?" *Frontiers in Microbiology* 2 (2011): 53. doi:10.3389/fmicb.2011.00053.

57. Gary B. Huffnagle, *The Probiotics Revolution*. (New York: Random House, 2008).

58. T. L. Carson et al., "Examining Social Influence on Participation and Outcomes among a Network of Behavioral Weight-Loss Intervention Enrollees," *Journal of Obesity* 2013 (2013) Article ID 480630.

59. Christakis and Fowler, "The Spread of Obesity in a Large Social Network Over 32 Years."

CHAPTER 8

1.   S. L. Teegarden and T. L. Bale, "Effects of Stress on Dietary Preference and Intake Are Dependent on Access and Stress Sensitivity," *Physiology & Behavior* 93, nos. 4–5 (March 18, 2008): 713–23.

2.   M. Siervo, J. C. Wells, and G. Cizza, "The Contribution of Psychosocial Stress to the Obesity Epidemic: An Evolutionary Approach," *Hormone and Metabolic Research* 41, no. 4 (April 2009): 261–70.

3.   J. Maniam and M. J. Morris, "Long-Term Postpartum Anxiety and Depression-Like Behavior in Mother Rats Subjected to Maternal Separation Are Ameliorated by Palatable High Fat Diet," *Behavioural Brain Research* 208, no. 1 (March 17, 2010): 72–79.

4.   Ibid.

5.   M. F. Dallman, "Stress-Induced Obesity and the Emotional Nervous System," *Trends in Endocrinology and Metabolism* 21, no. 3 (March 2010): 159–65.

6.   Dina Aronson, "Cortisol—Its Role in Stress, Inflammation, and Indications for Diet Therapy, *Today's Dietitian,* November 2009, 38, accessed April 5, 2013, http://www.todaysdietitian.com/newarchives/111609p38.shtml.

7.   E. Epel et al., "Stress May Add Bite to Appetite in Women: A Laboratory Study of Stress-Induced Cortisol and Eating Behavior," *Psychoneuroendocrinology* 26, no. 1 (January 2001): 37–49.

8.   L. E. Kuo et al., "Neuropeptide Y Acts Directly in the Periphery on Fat Tissue and Mediates Stress-Induced Obesity and Metabolic Syndrome," *Nature Medicine* 13, no. 7 (July 2007): 803–11

9.   M. Siervo, J. C. Wells, and G. Cizza, "The Contribution of Psychosocial Stress to the Obesity Epidemic: An Evolutionary Approach," *Hormone and Metabolic Research* 41, no. 4 (April 2009): 261–70.

10.   N. Pecoraro et al., "Chronic Stress Promotes Palatable Feeding, Which Reduces Signs of Stress: Feedforward and Feedback Effects of Chronic Stress," *Endocrinology* 145, no. 8 (August 2004): 3754–62.

11.   A. J. Tomiyama, M. F. Dallman, and E. S. Epel, "Comfort Food Is Comforting to Those Most Stressed: Evidence of the Chronic Stress Response Network in High Stress Women," *Psychoneuroendocrinology* 36, no. 10 (November 2011): 1513–19.

12.   M. S. Tryon, R. Decant, and K. D. Laugero, "Having Your Cake and Eating It Too: A Habit of Comfort Food May Link Chronic Social Stress Exposure and Acute Stress-Induced Cortisol Hyporesponsiveness," *Physiology & Behavior* 114–15 (March 15, 2013): 32–37. doi: 10.1016/j.physbeh.2013.02.018.

13.   Dallman, "Stress-Induced Obesity and the Emotional Nervous System."

14.   L. Schwabe and O. T. Wolf, "Stress Prompts Habit Behavior in Humans," *Journal of Neuroscience* 29, no. 22 (June 3, 2009): 7191–98.

15.   A. Arnsten, "Stress Signalling Pathways That Impair Prefrontal Cortex Structure and Function," *Nature Reviews. Neuroscience* 10, no. 6 (June 2009): 410–422. doi: 10.1038/nrn2648.

16. C. D. Conrad, "Chronic Stress-Induced Hippocampal Vulnerability: The Glucocorticoid Vulnerability Hypothesis," *Reviews in the Neurosciences* 19, no. 6 (2008): 395–411.

17. T. Lee et al., "Chronic Stress Selectively Reduces Hippocampal Volume in Rats: A Longitudinal Magnetic Resonance Imaging Study," *NeuroReport* 20, no. 17 (November 25, 2009): 1554–58.

18. Y. Kuperman et al., "Perifornical Urocortin-3 Mediates the Link between Stress-Induced Anxiety and Energy Homeostasis," *Proceedings of the National Academy of Sciences of the United States of America* 107, no. 18 (May 4, 2010): 8393–98.

19. M. Lutter et al., "The Orexigenic Hormone Ghrelin Defends Against Depressive Symtoms of Chronic Stress," *Nature Neuroscience* 11, no. 7 (July 2008): 752–53.

20. A. Lowden et al., "Eating and Shift Work-effects on habits, metabolism and performance," *Scandinavian Journal of Work, Environment & Health* 36, no. 2 (March 2010), 150–62.

21. A. J. Davidson et al., "Chronic Jet-Lag Increases Mortality in Aged Mice," *Current Biology* 16, no. 21 (November 7, 2006): R914–16.

22. M. E. Wilson et al., "Quantifying Food Intake in Socially Housed Monkeys: Social Status Effects on Caloric Consumption," *Physiology & Behavior* 94, no. 4 (July 5, 2008): 586–94.

23. J. O. Hill, J. C. Peters, "Environmental Contributions to the Obesity Epidemic," *Science* 280, no. 5368 (May 29, 1998): 1371–74.

24. M. Elovainio et al., "Socioeconomic Differences in Cardiometabolic Factors: Social Causation or Health-Related Selection? Evidence from the Whitehall II Cohort Study, 1991–2004," *American Journal of Epidemiology* 174, no. 7 (October 1, 2011): 779–89. doi: 10.1093/aje/kwr149.

25. E. J. Brunner, T. Chandola, and M. G. Marmot, "Prospective Effect of Job Strain on General and Central Obesity in the Whitehall II Study," *American Journal of Epidemiology* 165, no. 7 (April 1, 2007): 828–37.

26. A. Moles et al., "Psychosocial Stress Affects Energy Balance in Mice: Modulation by Social Status," *Psychoneuroendocrinology* 31, no. 5 (June 2006): 623–33.

27. A. W. Smith, A. Baum and R. R. Wing, "Stress and Weight Gain in Parents of Cancer Patients," *International Journal of Obesity* 29, no. 2 (February 2005): 244–50.

28. Moles et al., "Psychosocial Stress Affects Energy Balance in Mice: Modulation by Social Status."

29. J. Brodersen and Volkert Dirk Siersma, "Long-Term Psychosocial Consequences of False-Positive Screening Mammography," *Annals of Family Medicine* 11, no. 2 (March–April 2013): 106–15. doi:10.1370/afm.1466.

30. S. Cohen and D. Janicki-Deverts, "Who's Stressed? Distributions of Psychological Stress in the United States in Probability Samples from 1983, 2006,

and 2009," *Journal of Applied Social Psychology* 42, no. 6 (June 2012): 1320–34.

31. S. Cohen et al., "Cardiovascular and Behavioral Effects of Community Noise," *American Scientist* 69, no. 5, (September–Octobet 1981): 528–535.

32. H. Ising and C. Braun, "Acute and Chronic Endocrine Effects of Noise: Review of the Research Conducted at the Institute for Water, Soil and Air Hygiene," *Noise Health* 2, no. 7 (2000): 7–24.

33. A. C. Mcfarlane, "The Long-Term Costs of Traumatic Stress: Intertwined Physical and Psychological Consequences," *World Psychiatry* 9, no. 1 (February 2010): 3–10.

34. S. Maguen et al., "The Relationship between Body Mass Index and Mental Health among Iraq and Afghanistan Veterans," *Journal of General Medicine* 28, suppl. 2 (July 2013): S563–70.

35. S. J. Torres and C. A. Noeson, "Relationship between Stress, Eating Behavior, and Obesity," *Nutrition* 23 nos. 11–12 (November–December, 2007): 887–94.

36. M. D. Lieberman et al., "Putting Feelings Into Words: Affect Labeling Disrupts Amygdala Activity in Response to Affective Stimuli," *Psychological Science* 15, no. 5 (May 2007): 421–28.

37. J. M. Soares et al., "Stress-Induced Changes in Human Decision-Making Are Reversible," *Translational Psychiatry* 2, no. 7 (July 2012): e131.

38. Richard Carlson, *Don't Sweat the Small Stuff—and it's all small stuff* (New York: Hyperion, 1996).

39. Email comments from Mary Dallman, April 18, 2013.

40. James W. Pennebaker, *Writing to Heal: A Guided Journal for Recovering from Trauma and Emotional Upheaval.* (Oakland, CA: New Harbinger Publications, 2004).

41. Anne Lamott, *Bird by Bird: Some Instructions on Writing and Life* (New York: Anchor, 1995).

42. Judith Wurtman, *Managing Your Mind & Mood Through Food* (New York: Harper Perennial, 1988).

43. Ibid.

44. J. Liu et al., "Regular Breakfast Consumption Is Associated with Increased IQ in Kindergarten Children," *Early Human Development* 89, no. 4 (April 2013): 257–62. doi: 10.1016/j.earlhumdev.2013.01.006.

45. L. Desbonnet et al., "Effects of the Probiotic Bifidobacterium Infantis in the Maternal Separation Model of Depression," *Neuroscience* 170, no. 4 (November 10, 2010): 1179–88. doi: 10.1016/j.neuroscience.2010.08.005.

46. T. C. Goes et al., "Effect of Sweet Orange Aroma on Experimental Anxiety in Humans," *Journal of Alternative & Complementary Medicine* 18, no. 8 (August 2012): 798–804. doi: 10.1089/acm.2011.0551.

47. A. Tsatsoulis and S. Fountoulakis, "The Protective Role of Exercise on Stress System Dysregulation and Comorbidities," *Annals of the New York Academy of Sciences* 1083 (November 2006): 196–213.

48. Martin E. P. Seligman, *Learned Optimism* (New York: Alfred A. Knopf, 1991).

CHAPTER 9

1. S. Haley, "Sugar and Sweeteners Outlook," June 18, 2012, http://www.ers.usda.gov/media/816164/sssm286.pdf.

2. "Antibiotics and the Meat We Eat," *New York Times*, accessed April 6, 2013, http://www.nytimes.com/2013/03/28/opinion/antibiotics-and-the-meat-we-eat.html.

3. "World Health Day 2011: Urgent Action Necessary to Safeguard Drug Treatments," April 6, 2011, World Health Organization, February 1, 2012, http://www.who.int/mediacentre/news/releases/2011/whd_20110406/en/index.html.

4. Robert S. Lawrence, "The Rise of Antibiotic Resistance: Consequences of FDA's Inaction," *The Atlantic*, January 23, 2012, http://www.theatlantic.com/health/archive/2012/01/the-rise-of-antibiotic-resistance-consequences-of-fdas-inaction/251754.

5. F. Thuny et al., "Vancomycin Treatment of Infective Endocarditis Is Linked with Recently Acquired Obesity," *PLOS ONE* 5, no. 2 (February 10, 2010): e9074.

6. I. H. Rosenberg et al., "Infant and Child Enteritis-Malabsorption-Malnutrition: The Potential of Limited Studies with Low-Dose Antibiotic Feeding," *American Journal of Clinical Nutrition* 27, no. 3 (March 1974): 304–9.

7. B. R. Berends et al., "Human Health Hazards Associated with the Administration of Antimicrobials to Slaughter Animals. Part I. An Assessment of the Risks of Residues of Tetracyclines in Pork," *Veterinary Quarterly* 23, no. 1 (January 2001):2–10.

8. I. Dohoo et al., "A Meta-Analysis Review of the Effects of Recombinant Bovine Somatotropin: 1. Methodology and Effects on Production." *Canadian Journal of Veterinary Research* 67, no. 4 (October 1, 2003): 241–51, http://www.pubmedcentral.nih.gov/articlerender.fcgi?tool=pmcentrez&artid=280708.

9. Ibid.

10. Donald L. Barlett and James B. Steele, "Monsanto's Harvest of Fear,". *Vanity Fair*, 2008, accessed August 12, 2012, http://www.vanityfair.com/politics/features/2008/05/monsanto200805.

11. "Labeling & Standards," International Dairy Foods Association, http://www.idfa.org/key-issues/category/labeling--standards.

12. Bartlett and Steele, "Monsanto's Harvest of Fear."

13. I. Dohoo et al., "A Meta-Analysis Review of the Effects of Recombinant Bovine Somatotropin: 1. Methodology and Effects on Production." *Canadian Journal of Veterinary Research* 67, no. 4 (October 1, 2003): 241–51, http://www.pubmedcentral.nih.gov/articlerender.fcgi?tool=pmcentrez&artid=280708.

14. L. Q. Qin, K. He, J. Y. Xu, "Milk Consumption and Circulating Insulin-Like Growth Factor-I Level: A Systematic Literature Review," *International Journal of Food Sciences and Nutrition* 60, suppl. 7 (2009): 330–40.

15. S. A. Rosenzweig and H. S. Atreya, "Defining the Pathway to Insulin-Like Growth Factor System Targeting in Cancer," *Biochemical Pharmacology* 80, no. 8 (October 15, 2010): 1115–24.

16. B. C. Melnik, "Milk—The Promoter of Chronic Western Diseases." *Medical Hypotheses* 72, no. 6 (June 2009): 631–39.

17. Richard Laliberte, "Growth Hormones in Beef and Milk," *Weight Watchers.com,* accessed April 22, 2013, http://www.weightwatchers.com/util/art/index_art.aspx?tabnum=1&art_id=111911.

18. J. Vicini et al., "Survey of Retail Milk Composition As Affected by Label Claims Regarding Farm-Management Practices," *Journal of the American Dietetic Associaton* 108, no. 7 (July 2008): 1198–203.

19. J. Vicini et al., "Steroid Hormone Implants Used for Growth in Food-Producing Animals," Food and Drug Administration, http://www.fda.gov/AnimalVeterinary/SafetyHealth/ProductSafetyInformation/ucm055436.htm.

20. W. A. Kerr and J. E. Hobbs, "The North American-European Dispute over Beef Produced Using Growth Hormones: A Major Test for the New International Trade Regime," accessed April 8, 2013, http://are.berkeley.edu/courses/EEP131/old_files/HormonesKerrandHobbs.pdf.

21. Richard Laliberte, "Growth Hormones in Beef and Milk," *Weight Watchers.com*, accessed April 22, 2013, http://www.weightwatchers.com/util/art/index_art.aspx?tabnum=1&art_id=111911.

22. L. N. Vandenberg et al., "Hormones and Endocrine-Disrupting Chemicals: Low-Dose Effects and Nonmonotonic Dose Responses," *Endocrine Reviews* 33, no. 3 (June 2012): 378–455.

23. Marla Cone, "Low Doses, Big Effects: Scientists Seek 'Fundamental Changes' in Testing, Regulation of Hormone-Like Chemicals," *Environmental Health News*, March 15, 2012, http://www.environmentalhealthnews.org/ehs/news/2012/low-doses-big-effects.

24. Buck Levin, *Environmental Nutrition*(HingePin Integrative Learning Materials:1999).

25. "Sugar and Sweeteners: Background," USDA Economic Research Service, accessed October 31, 2013, last updated October 9, 2012, http://www.ers.usda.gov/topics/crops/sugar-sweeteners/background.aspx#.UnNZij78K00.

26. Luc Tappy and Kim-Anne Lê, " Metabolic Effects of Fructose and the Worldwide Increase in Obesity," *Physiological Reviews* 90, no. 1 (January 2010): 23–46. doi:10.1152/physrev.00019.2009

27. K. L. Teff et al., "Dietary Fructose Reduces Circulating Insulin and Leptin, Attenuates Postprandial Suppression of Ghrelin, and Increases Triglycerides in Women," *Journal of Clinical Endocrinology & Metabolism* 89, no. 6 (June 2004): 2963–72.

28. A. Shapiro et al., "Fructose-Induced Leptin Resistance Exacerbates Weight Gain in Response to Subsequent High-Fat Feeding," *American Journal of Physiology - Regulatory, Integrative and Comparative Physiology* 295, no. 5 (November 2008): R1370–75.

29. Teff et al., "Dietary Fructose Reduces Circulating Insulin."

30. S. H. Cha et al., "Differential Effects of Central Fructose and Glucose on Hypothalamic Malonyl–Coa and Food Intake," *Proceedings of the National Academy of Sciences of the United States of America* 105, no. 44 (November 2008): 16871–75. doi:10.1073/pnas.0809255105.

31. K. A. Page et al., "Effects of Fructose vs. Glucose on Regional Cerebral Blood Flow in Brain Regions Involved with Appetite and Reward Pathways," *Journal of the American Medical Association* 309, no. 1 (January 2, 2013): 63–70. doi: 10.1001/jama.2012.116975.

32. H. Jürgens et al., "Consuming Fructose-Sweetened Beverages Increases Body Adiposity in Mice," *Obesity Research* 13, no. 7 (July 2005): 1146–56.

33. C. L. Cox et al., "Consumption of Fructose-Sweetened Beverages for 10 Weeks Reduces Net Fat Oxidation and Energy Expenditure in Overweight/Obese Men and Women," *European Journal of Clinical Nutrition* 66, no. 2 (February 2012):201–8.

34. B. Stavric et al., "Effect of Fructose Administration on Serum Urate Levels in the Uricase Inhibited Rat," *Experientia* 32, no. 2 (March 15, 1976): 373–74.

35. Luc Tappy and Kim-Anne Lê, "Metabolic Effects of Fructose and the Worldwide Increase in Obesity," *Physiological Reviews* 90, no. 1 (January 2010): 23–46. doi:10.1152/physrev.00019.2009.

36. Q. Shao and K. V. Chin, "Survey of American Food Trends and the Growing Obesity Epidemic," *Nutrition Research and Practice* 5, no. 3 (June 2011): 253–59.

37. Andrew Pollack, "After Loss, the Fight to Label Modified Food Continues," *New York Times*, November 7, 2012, accessed November 8, 2012, http://www.nytimes.com/2012/11/08/business/california-bid-to-label-genetically-modified-crops.html?hpw.

38. Greg Critser, *Fat Land* (New York: Penguin Books, 2003).

39. L. R. Vartanian, M. B. Schwartz, and K. D. Brownell, "Effects of Soft Drink Consumption on Nutrition and Health: A Systematic Review and Meta-Analysis," *American Journal of Public Health* 97, no. 4 (April 2007): 667–75.

40. R. A. Forshee, P. A. Anderson, and M. L. Storey, "Sugar-Sweetened Beverages and Body Mass Index in Children and Adolescents: A Meta-Analysis," *American Journal of Clinical Nutrition* 87, no. 6 (June 2008): 1662–71.

41. L. K. Midtbø et al., "Intake of Farmed Atlantic Salmon Fed Soybean Oil Increases Insulin Resistance and Hepatic Lipid Accumulation in Mice," *PLOS ONE* 8, no. 1 (January 2013): e53094. doi: 10.1371/journal.pone.0053094.

42. M. L. de Lemos, "Effects of Soy Phytoestrogens Genistein and Daidzein

on Breast Cancer Growth," *Annals of Pharmacotherapy* 35, no. 9 (September 2001): 1118–21.

43. N. Moussavi, V. Gavino, and O. Receveur, "Could the Quality of Dietary Fat, and Not Just Its Quantity, Be Related to Risk of Obesity?" *Obesity* (Silver Spring, MD) 16, no. 1 (January 2008): 7–15.

44. "Accomplishments," Center for Science in the Public Interest, http://www.cspinet.org/about/accomplishments.

45. K. Kavanagh et al., "Trans Fat Diet Induces Abdominal Obesity and Changes in Insulin Sensitivity in Monkeys," *Obesity* (Silver Spring, MD) 15, no. 7 (July 2007): 1675–84.

46. M. Hermanussen et al., "Obesity, Voracity, and Short Stature: The Impact of Glutamate on the Regulation of Appetite," *European Journal of Clinical Nutrition* 60, no. 1 (January 2005): 25–31.

47. "Wegmans Potato Chips, Barbecue," Fooducate, http://www.fooducate.com/app#page=product&id=2ABEFCB8-E112-11DF-A102-FEFD45A4D471.

48. M. Hermanussen et al., "Obesity, Voracity, and Short Stature: The Impact of Glutamate on the Regulation of Appetite," *European Journal of Clinical Nutrition* 60, no. 1 (January 2005): 25–31.

49. K. He et al., "Association of Monosodium Glutamate Intake with Overweight in Chinese Adults: The INTERMAP Study," *Obesity* (Silver Spring, MD) 16, no. 8 (August 2008): 1875–80.

50. K. He et al., "Consumption of Monosodium Glutamate in Relation to Incidence of Overweight in Chinese Adults: China Health and Nutrition Survey (CHNS)," *American Journal of Clinical Nutrition* 93, no. 6 (June 2011): 1328–36.

51. M. Hermanussen and J. A. Tresguerres, "Does High Glutamate Intake Cause Obesity?" *Journal of Pediatric Endocrinology & Metabolism* 16, no. 7 (September 2003): 965–68.

52. Q. Yang, "Gain Weight by 'Going Diet?' Artificial Sweeteners and the Neurobiology of Sugar Cravings: Neuroscience 2010," *Yale Journal of Biology and Medicine* 83, no. 2 (June 2010): 101–8

53. Food http://www.foodfacts.com/ Accessed April 10, 2013.

54. Yang, "Gain Weight by 'Going Diet?'"

55. R. D. Mattes and B. M. Popkin, "Nonnutritive Sweetener Consumption in Humans: Effects on Appetite and Food Intake and Their Putative Mechanisms," *American Journal of Clinical Nutrition* 89, no. 1 (January 2009): 1–14. doi: 10.3945/ajcn.2008.26792.

56. Yang, "Gain Weight by 'Going Diet?'"

57. M. A. Mohamed and A. S. Ammar, "Quantitative Analysis of Phthalates Plasticizers in Traditional Egyptian Foods (Koushary and Foul Medams), Black Tea, Instant Coffee and Bottled Waters by Solid Phase Extraction-Capillary Gas Chromatography-Mass Spectroscopy," *American Journal of Food Technology* 3, no. 5 (2008): 341–46. doi: 10.3923/ajft.2008.341.346.

58. M. J. Silva et al., "Urinary Levels of Seven Phthalate Metabolites in the

U.S. Population from the National Health and Nutrition Examination Survey (NHANES) 1999–2000," *Environmental Health Perspectives* 112, no. 3 (March 2004): 331–38.

59. "Phthalates," Consumer Product Safety Commission, https://www.cpsc.gov/phthalates.

60. S. H. Swan et al., "Prenatal Phthalate Exposure and Reduced Masculine Play in Boys," *International Journal of Andrology* 33, no. 2 (April 2010): 259–69.

61. R. W. Stahlhut et al., "Concentrations of Urinary Phthalate Metabolites Are Associated with Increased Waist Circumference and Insulin Resistance in Adult U.S. Males," *Environmental Health Perspectives* 115, no. 6 (June 2007): 876–82.

62. Lindsey Partos, "Parabens: Food Authority Proposes Limit for Food Preservative," *FoodNavigator.com*, September 30, 2004, accessed April 22, 2013. http://www.foodnavigator.com/Legislation/Parabens-food-authority-proposes-limit-for-food-preservative.

63. M. A. Elobeid and D. B. Allison, "Putative Environmental-Endocrine Disruptors and Obesity: A Review," *Current Opinion in Endocrinology, Diabetes & Obesity* 15, no. 5 (October 2008): 403–8. doi: 10.1097/MED.0b013e32830ce95c.

64. Center for Science in the Public Interest, http://www.cspinet.org.

65. Marion Nestle, *Food Politics* (Los Angeles: University of California Press, 2003).

66. "National Organic Program," USDA Argicultural Marketing Service, http://www.ams.usda.gov/AMSv1.0/ams.fetchTemplateData.do?template=TemplateC&navID=NationalOrganicProgram&leftNav=NationalOrganicProgram&page=NOPConsumers&description=Consumers&acct=nopgeninfo.

67. "Food News," Environmental Working Group, accessed April 8, 2013, http://www.ewg.org/foodnews/ Accessed April 8, 2013.

68. "Industry Statistics and Projected Growth," Organic Trade Association, http://www.ota.com/organic/mt/business.html.

69. S. Haley, "Sugar and Sweeteners Outlook," United States Department of Agriculture, June 18, 2012, http://www.ers.usda.gov/media/816164/sssm286.pdf.

70. Jonathan Landsman, *Natural Health 365*, December 12, 2011, http://www.naturalhealth365.com/tag/glutamic-acid

71. "Learn about Global Efforts to Reduce Waste from Disposable Products," accessed April 2, 2012, http://reusablebags.com/learn-more/top-facts/trends-from-around-the-world.

72. J. L. Carwile et al., "Polycarbonate Bottle Use and Urinary Bisphenol A Concentrations," *Environmental Health Perspectives* 117, no. 9 (September 2009): 1368–72. doi: 10.1289/ehp.0900604.

CHAPTER 10

1.   U. Albrecht, "Timing to Perfection: The Biology of Central and Peripheral Circadian Clocks," *Neuron* 74, no. 2 (April 2012): 246–60.

2.   I. N. Karatsoreos et al., "Disruption of Circadian Clocks Has Ramifications for Metabolism, Brain, and Behavior," *Proceedings of the National Academy of Sciences* 108, no. 4 (January 25, 2011):1657–62. doi: 10.1073/pnas.1018375108.

3.   Frank B. Hu, *Obesity Epidemiology* (New York: Oxford University Press, 2008).

4.   National Sleep Foundation, *2003 Sleep in America Poll*, March 10, 2003, http://www.sleepfoundation.org/sites/default/files/2003SleepPollExecSumm .pdf.

5.   National Sleep Foundation, *2008 Sleep in America Poll*, MArch 2, 2008, http://www.sleepfoundation.org/sites/default/files/2008%20POLL%20SOF.PDF.

6.   National Sleep Foundation, *2005 Sleep in America Poll*, March 29, 2005, http://www.sleepfoundation.org/sites/default/files/2005_summary_of_findings .pdf.

7.   K. L. Knutson et al., "Trends in the Prevalence of Short Sleepers in the USA: 1975–2006," *Sleep* 33, no. 1 (January 2010): 37–45.

8.   E. Kronholm et al., "Trends in Self-Reported Sleep Duration and Insomnia-Related Symptoms in Finland from 1972 to 2005: A Comparative Review and Re-Analysis of Finnish Population Samples," *Journal of Sleep Research* 17, no. 1 (March 2008): 54–62.

9.   R. A. Rowshan et al., "Thirty-Six-Year Secular Trends in Sleep Duration and Sleep Satisfaction, and Associations with Mental Stress and Socioeconomic Factors – Results of the Population Study of Women in Gothenburg, Sweden," *Journal of Sleep Research* 19, no. 3 (September 2010): 496–503. doi: 10.1111/j.1365-2869.2009.00815.x.

10.   National Sleep Foundation, *2011 Sleep in America Poll*, 2011, http://www.sleepfoundation.org/sites/default/files/sleepinamericapoll/SIAP_2011 _Summary_of_Findings.pdf

11.   Ismat Sarah Mangla, "Cheap Ways to Get More Sleep," *Money Magazine*, April 19, 2012. Accessed online April 12, 2013.

12.   F. J. Zinnermann and J. F. Bell, "Associations of Television Content Type and Obesity in Children," *American Journal of Public Health* 100, no. 2 (February 2010): 334–40. doi: 10.2105/AJPH.2008.155119.

13.   N. Cotugna, "TV Ads on Saturday Morning Children's Programming—What's New?" *Journal of Nutrition Education* 20, no. 3 (May–June 1988): 125–27.

14.   K. Harrison and A. L. Marske, "Nutritional Content of Foods Advertised during the Television Programs Children Watch Most," *American Journal of Public Health* 95, no. 9 (September 2005): 1568–74.

15.   Juliet B. Schor, *Born to Buy: The Commercialized Child and the New Consumer Culture* (New York: Scribner; 2004).

16. Zinnermann and Bell, "Associations of Television Content Type and Obesity in Children."

17. Ibid.

18. L. H. Epstein et al., "A Randomized Trial of the Effects of Reducing Television Viewing and Computer Use on Body Mass Index in Young Children," *Archives of Pediatrics and Adolescent Medicine* 162, no. 3 (March 2008): 239–45. doi: 10.1001/archpediatrics.2007.45.

19. E. A. Vandewater, M. S. Shim, and A. G. Caplovitz, "Linking Obesity and Activity Level with Children's Television and Video Game Use," *Journal of Adolescence* 27, no. 1 (February 2004): 71–85.

20. C. Vandelanotte et al., "Associations of Leisure-Time Internet and Computer Use with Overweight and Obesity, Physical Activity and Sedentary Behaviors: Cross-Sectional Study," *Journal of Medical Internet Research* 11, no. 3 (July 27, 2009): e28.

21. H. M. al-Hazzaa et al., "Physical Activity, Sedentary Behaviors and Dietary Habits among Saudi Adolescents Relative to Age, Gender and Region," *International Journal of Behavioral Nutrition and Physical Activity* 8 (December 21, 2011): 140.

22. National Sleep Foundation, *2011 Sleep in America Poll*, 2011, http://www.sleepfoundation.org/sites/default/files/sleepinamericapoll/SIAP_2011_Summary_of_Findings.pdf

23. F. P. Cappuccio et al., "Meta-Analysis of Short Sleep Duration and Obesity in Children and Adults," *Sleep* 31, no. 5 (May 1, 2008): 619–26.

24. S. R. Patel and F. B. Hu, "Sleep Deprivation" in F. Hu, ed., *Obesity Epidemiology* (New York: Oxford University Press, 2008), 320–41.

25. C. R. Moreno et al., "Short Sleep Is Associated with Obesity among Truck Drivers," *Chronobiology International* 23, no. 6 (2006): 1295–303.

26. N. D. Kohatsu et al., "Sleep Duration and Body Mass Index in a Rural Population," *Archives of Internal Medicine* 166, no. 16 (September 18, 2006): 1701–5.

27. H. Shigeta et al., "Lifestyle, Obesity, and Insulin Resistance," *Diabetes Care* 24, no. 3 (March 2001): 608.

28. M. Cournot et al., "Environmental Factors Associated with Body Mass Index in a Population of Southern France," *European Journal of Cardiovascular Prevention and Rehabilitation* 11, no. 4 (August 2004): 291–97.

29. J. Vioque, A. Torres, J. Quiles, "Time Spent Watching Television, Sleep Duration and Obesity in Adults Living in Valencia, Spain," *International Journal of Obesity and Related Metabolic Disorders* 24, no. 12 (December 2000): 1683–88.

30. R. D. Vorona et al., "Overweight and Obese Patients in a Primary Care Population Report Less Sleep Than Patients with a Normal Body Mass Index," *Archives of Internal Medicine* 165, no. 1 (January 10, 2005): 25–30.

31. M. Singh et al., "The Association between Obesity and Short Sleep Duration: A Population-Based Study," *Journal of Clinical Sleep Medicine* 1, no. 4 (October 15, 2005): 357–63.

32. L. Hale and D. P. Do, "Racial Differences in Self-Reports of Sleep Duration in a Population-Based Study," *Sleep* 30, no. 9 (September 1, 2007): 1096–103.

33. "Health of Black or African American non-Hispanic Population," Centers for Disease Control and Prevention, last modified August 5, 2013, http://www.cdc.gov/nchs/faststats/black_health.htm

34. S. R. Patel et al., "Association between Reduced Sleep and Weight Gain in Women," *American Journal of Epidemiology* 164, no. 10 (November 15, 2006): 947–54.

35. J. Gangwisch and S. Heymsfield, "Sleep Deprivation As a Risk Factor for Obesity: Results Based on the NHANESI," *North American Association for the Study of Obesity* (NAASO). 2004. 2004 Abstract no. 42-OR:A11

36. G. Hasler et al., "The Association between Short Sleep Duration and Obesity in Young Adults: A 13-Year Prospective Study," *Sleep* 27, no. 4 (June 15, 2004): 661–66.

37. S. Taheri et al., "Short Sleep Duration Is Associated with Reduced Leptin, Elevated Ghrelin, and Increased Body Mass Index," *Public Library of Science Medicine* 1, no. 3 (December 2004): e62.

38. R. Leproult, E. van Cauter, "Role of Sleep and Sleep Loss in Hormonal Release and Metabolism," *Endocrine Development* 17 (2010): 11–21.

39. E. Locard et al., "Risk Factors of Obesity in a Five Year Old Population. Parental Versus Environmental Factors," *International Journal of Obesity and Related Metabolic Disorders* 16, no. 10 (October 1992): 721–29.

40. R. von Kries et al., "Reduced Risk for Overweight and Obesity in 5- and 6-Y-Old Children by Duration of Sleep—A Cross-Sectional Study," *International Journal of Obesity and Related Metabolic Disorders* 26, no. 5 (May 2002): 710–16.

41. M. Sekine et al., "A Dose-Response Relationship between Short Sleeping Hours and Childhood Obesity: Results of the Toyama Birth Cohort Study," *Child: Care, Health and Development* 28, no. 2 (March 2002): 163–70.

42. W. S. Agras et al., "Risk Factors for Childhood Overweight: A Prospective Study from Birth to 9.5 Years," *Journal of Pediatrics* 145, no. 1 (July 2004): 20–25.

43. H. Sugimori et al., "Analysis of Factors That Influence Body Mass Index from Ages 3 to 6 Years: A Study Based on the Toyama Cohort Study," *Pediatrics International* 46, no. 3 (June 2004): 302–10.

44. N. K. Gupta et al., "Is Obesity Associated with Poor Sleep Quality in Adolescents?" *American Journal of Human Biology* 14, no. 6 (November–December 2002): 762–68.

45. Hu, *Obesity Epidemiology.*

46. S. Taheri, "Sleep and Metabolism: Bringing Pieces of the Jigsaw Together," *Sleep Medicine Reviews* 11, no. 3 (June 2007): 159–62.

47. S. M. Schmid et al., "Short-Term Sleep Loss Decreases Physical Activity Under Free-Living Conditions but Does Not Increase Food Intake Under Time-Deprived Laboratory Conditions in Healthy Men," *American Journal of Clinical Nutrition* 90, no. 6 (December 2009): 1476–82.

48. S. R. Patel et al., "Association between Reduced Sleep and Weight Gain in Women," *American Journal of Epidemiology* 164, no. 10 (November 15, 2006): 947–54.

49. G. Savourey and J. Bittel, "Cold Thermoregulatory Changes Induced by Sleep Deprivation in Men," *European Journal of Applied Physiology and Occupational Physiology* 69, no. 3 (1994): 216–20.

50. O. M. Buxton et al., "Adverse Metabolic Consequences in Humans of Prolonged Sleep Restriction Combined with Circadian Disruption," *Science Translational Medicine* 4, no 129 (April 11, 2012): 129ra43.

51. R. R. Markwald et al., "Impact of Insufficient Sleep on Total Daily Energy Expenditure, Food Intake, and Weight Gain," *Proceedings of the National Academy of Sciences* 110, no. 14 (April 2, 2013): 5695–700. doi: 10.1073/pnas.1216951110.

52. Buxton et al., "Adverse Metabolic Consequences in Humans of Prolonged Sleep Restriction Combined with Circadian Disruption."

53. E. van Cauter and K. Spiegel, "Sleep As a Mediator of the Relationship between Socioeconomic Status and Health: A Hypothesis," *Annals of the New York Academy of Sciences* 896 (1999): 254–61.

54. K. L. Knutson et al., "The Metabolic Consequences of Sleep Deprivation," *Sleep Medicine Reviews* 11, no. 3 (June 2007): 163–78.

55. K. Spiegel, R. Leproult, and E. van Cauter, "Impact of Sleep Debt on Metabolic and Endocrine Function," *Lancet* 354, no. 9188 (October 23, 1999): 1435–39.

56. K. Spiegel et al., "Leptin Levels Are Dependent on Sleep Duration: Relationships with Sympathovagal Balance, Carbohydrate Regulation, Cortisol, and Thyrotropin," *The Journal of Clinical Endocrinology & Metabolism* 89, no. 11 (November 2004): 5762–71.

57. Knutson et al., "Metabolic Consequences."

58. Van Cauter E et al., "Reciprocal Interactions between the GH Axis and Sleep," *Growth Hormone & IGF Research* 14, suppl. A (June 2004): S10–7.

59. C. A. Everson and W. R. Crowley, "Reductions in Circulating Anabolic Hormones Induced by Sustained Sleep Deprivation in Rats," *American Journal of Physiology: Endocrinology and Metabolism* 26, no. 6 (June 2004): E1060–70.

60. S. Taheri et al., "Short Sleep Duration Is Associated with Reduced Leptin, Elevated Ghrelin, and Increased Body Mass Index," *Public Library of Science Medicine* 1, no. 3 (December 2004): e62.

61. K. Spiegel et al., "Brief Communication: Sleep Curtailment in Healthy Young Men Is Associated with Decreased Leptin Levels, Elevated Ghrelin Levels, and Increased Hunger and Appetite," *Annals of Internal Medicine* 141, no. 11 (December 7, 2004): 846–50.

62. K. Spiegel et al., "Brief Communication: Sleep Curtailment in Healthy Young Men."

63. S. Taheri et al., "Short Sleep Duration."

64. Spiegel et al., "Brief Communication: Sleep Curtailment in Healthy Young Men."

65. M. Pedrazzoli et al., "Increased Hypocretin-1 Levels in Cerebrospinal Fluid After REM Sleep Deprivation," *Brain Research* 995, no. 1 (January 2, 2004): 1–6.

66. S. M. Holm et al., "Reward-Related Brain Function and Sleep in Pre/Early Pubertal and Mid/Late Pubertal Adolescents," *Journal of Adolescent Health* 45, no. 4 (October 2009): 326–34.

67. N. Tsujino and T. Sakurai, "Orexin/Hypocretin: A Neuropeptide at the Interface of Sleep, Energy Homeostasis, and Reward System," *Pharmacological Reviews* 61, no. 2 (June 2009): 162–76.

68. A. Lacquaniti et al., "Obestatin: An Interesting but Controversial Gut Hormone," *Annals of Nutrition & Metabolism* 59, nos. 2–4 (2011): 193–99.

69. A. J. Stunkard and S. Messick, "The Three-Factor Eating Questionnaire to Measure Dietary Restraint, Disinhibition and Hunger," *Journal of Psychosomatic Research* 29, no. 1 (1985): 71–83.

70. J. P. Chaput et al., "The Association between Short Sleep Duration and Weight Gain Is Dependent on Disinhibited Eating Behavior in Adults," *Sleep* 34, no. 10 (October 1, 2011): 1291–97.

71. A. V. Nedeltcheva et al., "Sleep Curtailment Is Accompanied by Increased Intake of Calories from Snacks," *American Journal of Clinical Nutrition* 89, no. 1 (January 2009): 126–33.

72. E. J. Bryant, N. A. King, and J. E. Blundell, "Disinhibition: Its Effects on Appetite and Weight Regulation," *Obesity Reviews* 9, no. 5 (September 2008): 409–19.

73. A. Weiss et al., "The Association of Sleep Duration to Adolescents' Fat and Carbohydrate Consumption," *Sleep* 33, no. 9 (September 1, 2010):1201–9.

74. N. Goel et al., "Circadian Rhythm Profiles in Women with Night Eating Syndrome," *Journal of Biological Rhythms* 24, no. 1 (February 2009): 85–94.

75. Ibid.

76. G. Cizza et al., "Treatment of Obesity with Extension of Sleep Duration: A Randomized, Prospective, Controlled Trial," *Clinical Trials* (London, England) 7, no. 3 (June 2010): 274–85.

77. Ismat Sarah Mangla, "Cheap Ways to Get More Sleep," *Money Magazine* April 19, 2012, accessed online April 12, 2013, http://money.cnn.com/2012/04/19/pf/sleep-loss.moneymag.

78. S. Guy, A. Ratzki-Leewing, and F. Gwadry-Sridhar, "Moving beyond the Stigma: Systematic Review of Video Games and Their Potential to Combat Obesity," *International Journal of Hypertension* 2011 (2011): 1–13.

79. Ibid.

80. M. A. Napolitano et al., "Using Facebook and Text Messaging to Deliver a Weight Loss Program to College Students," *Obesity* (Silver Spring, MD) 21, no. 1 (January 2013): 25–31.

81. R. A. Rowshan et al., "Thirty-Six-Year Secular Trends in Sleep Duration and Sleep Satisfaction, and Associations with Mental Stress and Socioeconomic Factors – Results of the Population Study of Women in Gothenburg, Sweden," *Journal of Sleep Research* 19, no. 3 (September 2010): 496–503. doi: 10.1111/j.1365-2869.2009.00815.x.

82. B. Dickerman and J. Liu, "Does Current Scientific Evidence Support a Link between Light at Night and Breast Cancer among Female Night-Shift Nurses? Review of Evidence and Implications for Occupational and Environmental Health Nurses," *Workplace Health & Safety* 60, no. 6 (June 2012): 273–81. doi: 10.3928/21650799-20120529-06.

83. K. C. Allison et al., "Cognitive Behavior Therapy for Night Eating Syndrome: A Pilot Study," *American Journal of Psychotherapy* 64, no. 1 (2010): 91–106.

AFTERWORD

1. B. M. Popkin, L. S. Adair, and S. W. Ng, "NOW AND THEN: The Global Nutrition Transition: The Pandemic of Obesity in Developing Countries," *Nutrition Reviews* 70, no. 1 (January 2012): 3–21.

2. J. Ensor, "Cookery Lessons Back on the School Menu," *The Telegraph*, February 10, 2013, http://www.telegraph.co.uk/education/9859474/cookery-lessons-back-on-the-school-menu.html.

3. "Masadar City," *Wikipedia*, last modified September 12, 2013, http://en.wikipedia.org/wiki/Masdar_City

INDEX

· · · ·

X

Xbox 14, 101, 225

Y

Yale University 134, 204, 206, 212
Yale University School of Medicine 204
Yang, Qing 212

Yerkes National Primate Research Center, Emory University 182
yoga 50

Z

ziprasidone 46, 49
zonisamide 51

ACKNOWLEDGMENTS

· · · ·

GLOBESITY EMERGED FROM THE WORK OF scientists, scholars, dietitians, health care workers and public health activists in the field of obesity. Their dedicated pursuit of solutions to this pandemic moved me to distill science into a clear and urgent message.

I thank them for sharing generously across databases and the web, especially PubMed, a National Institutes of Health platform and gift from the citizens of the United States. Proximity to a medical library with open doors is no longer a requirement for scientific inquiry. Ideas can take shape and gather ballast in any village on earth thanks to this free flow of digital data and argument.

Egypt has been profound in my education. I lived through revolutions yet watched as obesity—which will kill more than civil unrest—swept a populace unable to pay the high costs of diabetes and other chronic diseases. I thank the kind people of Egypt for the warmest of welcomes and wish them the future they deserve. Inshallah.

Special appreciation goes out to the many researchers involved in "Ten Putative Contributors to the Obesity Epidemic," an influential body of work that insisted we look at new reasons for obesity.

I am particularly indebted to the distinguished Frank Hu, editor and major contributor to *Obesity Epidemiology*, a text of great importance and source of much background for my book.

Of significant note also are those scientists who reviewed sections of the book and contributed thoughtful commentary and critique:

Rosane Ness-Abramof, Retha Newbold, Russ Lopez, Barbara Rolls, Nikhil Dhurandhar, and Mary F. Dallman. Their creative and enduring exploration into drugs, pollutants, built environments, behavior, infections, and stress has led to discovery of negative health outcomes including obesity. Their generous responses prove that the excitement of shared learning lives on beyond commercial forces.

I owe much to my editors and all those at Cedar Fort. Haley Miller shaped the manuscript with an expert eye and astute intelligence. Whitney Lindsley fashioned the final book with all its quirks and endnotes using creativity and skill.

Family is all. I thank my husband. And my children. They give me joy.

I thank my dear father, Herbert, who lives with optimism and compassion. I am also grateful for my six brothers and sisters and their families with whom I travel through this life. I have been blessed.

With my husband's big family as well, I have extended that good fortune.

And to my brother Steve and my mother, Marcella, inspirations always: you both possessed the gifts of curiosity and wonder. I think you would have liked my questions here.

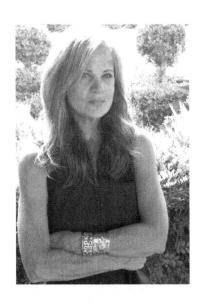

ABOUT THE AUTHOR

. . . .

REGISTERED DIETITIAN CLARE FLEISHMAN HAS worked in clinical, community and corporate settings globally to spread the message of good nutrition. She has published widely: *International Herald Tribune*, *Los Angeles Times*, the *Boston Globe*, the *Washington Post*, the *Philadelphia Inquirer*, *Weight Watchers Magazine*, and *Nutrition Forum*, among others. Her articles explore health issues in every vein: from diabetes to air pollution to fasting during Ramadan. Clare lives in Cairo, Egypt, where she counsels many patients struggling with obesity.

0   26575 12968   7